The Golden Egg

The Story of Our Miracle Baby

Debra L. Franco

Elias J. Franco

D&E Associates

Tampa, Florida

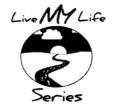

ACKNOWLEDGEMENT

We would like to thank Dr. David and Dr. Wayne for their tireless dedication in the pursuit of new technological advances for infertility, regardless of the critics and adversity they face each day in their profession.

Our sincere thanks also to Dr. Eric for his compassion, patience and dedication to the health and safety of both mother and child.

And, finally to the staff of Memorial Hospital in Hollywood, Florida, especially the doctors and nurses of the neonatal unit, for taking such good care of our miracle baby and sending her home happy and healthy.

DEDICATIONS

She Said...

This book is dedicated with oceans of love to my husband, Eli. His love, wisdom, humor and strength have inspired me to be the best that I can be. And to Shannon, Buddy and Madison who rock my world and are a constant source of light in my life. They each bring me bundles full of happiness each in their unique way. And, finally to Janet, Judy, Tia Beca and Lorna, my Forever Friends. I love you guys!

He Said...

Different people impact your life in different ways. To those special people in my life, I confess the following:

To Mom and Dad, I again say thank you for raising me the way you did, and for always being supportive and understanding.

To my sister Marilyn, thanks for helping out with the shots and 'injecting' the lucky booster.

To Shannon and Buddy, thanks for giving me an early preview on parenthood.

To Wayne, thanks for being a friend as well as a boss during those tumultuous times.

And to Debbie, my love, thanks for asking me to dance that October night, and for convincing me that "four" was a charm!

They Said...

And, to all the couples who think they can't have a child of their own: PERSEVERE. BELIEVE IN MIRACLES. They do come true.

Chapter One
The Infamous Dance

She Said...

I'd seen him a couple of times at Cadillac Jacks . . . an "old time" club we frequented on Wednesday and Friday nights. *Everyone* went there. We "hung out" there, my friends and I. It was a great place to dance away the night, have a few drinks and forget the stress in your life. We always seemed to meet nice people there and our circle of friends grew bigger and bigger. We got to know the bartenders and the waiters and before long, it felt like home. It was our place to go, meet and greet.

Eli always hung out on the "other side" of the circular shaped

1

dance floor. Every time I saw him in there, I thought he was sooooo cute. He had the most gorgeous eyes I had ever seen. Big, brown, almond-shaped, doe eyes. We made eye contact once or twice but that was it. Neither one of us ever took it any further because he was on "his side" and I was on the cool side! Besides, I wasn't looking for anything or anybody. I just wanted to dance and have fun. If someone asked me to dance, I would dance once or twice with him and then move on. My girlfriends were the same way. We all came together and we left together . . . with no extra guys tagging along.

On Wednesday night, the 28th of October, 1987 I walked into Cadillac Jacks . . . feeling great. Of course I had no idea that this night was predestined fate in the works, and that it would change the rest of my life. My planned-out, well-organized life! I looked hot and I knew it! Tight jeans and a cropped blouse with a sexy peek-a-boo back. I was even having a *Great Hair Day!* Sometimes you just know you're going to have a terrific time no matter where you go or what you do. This was definitely my night! I found my crowd of usual friends, grabbed a glass of wine and started scanning the place for familiar dance partners. Cadillac Jacks was a two-level building, the dance floor and two bars on the first level and booths and tables on the second level. We were eyeing the crowd from the second level when

2

I noticed that the cute, doe-eyed guy was on "my side" of the bar. He was usually with a tall guy wearing glasses when he came in, and sure enough his friend was right there with him.

I grabbed my girlfriend and said: "Look, there's that adorable guy . . . let's go down and stand over there. Maybe he'll ask me to dance."

She took one look at him and said: "I'm going to ask him to dance!"

"No way, I saw him first!" I replied.

"Okay, then *I dare you to ask him to dance* and if you don't, I will," she said. I hate dares and I hate to ask guys to dance. No way. She kept taunting me with her dares and when I saw he was tapping his feet to the music, I thought, well maybe he'll dance. As much as I disliked asking someone to dance, off I went . . . not feeling too confident despite the way I looked. Tap, tap on the shoulder.

"Um, excuse me, but would you like to dance?" (Oh my, am I really doing this?)

"No thanks, I don't like this song. Maybe another song. I'll come and get you when I'm ready to dance," he smugly told me.

To say I was humiliated is mild. I was devastated. Crushed. I knew I should never have asked. I hate asking guys to dance. They get so smug about it. They get this stupid little smile on their faces

3

as if they're making up for all the times *they* got turned down by some girl. And this guy was no different. Geez, did I feel like a total fool. *Never again.* Bet on it. I had to think quickly in order to cover my humiliation at being turned down, especially since my crowd was watching and they KNEW how much I hated doing what I got conned into doing. I was glad it was dark and this guy couldn't see my red face. So I said to him: "Buddy, now if you want to dance with me, you're going to have to get down on one knee and beg!" See ya.

I went back upstairs, humble but triumphant. At least I got the last word. As time passed and the music played on, my cheeks eventually returned to their normal color and I started feeling better after my bout of rejection. When I had the nerve to look down onto the first level, I saw the doe-eyed guy waving at me to come back down to where he was still standing with his friend. I thought, *what nerve, what an ego this guy has.* I can't believe he really thinks he can turn me down and then just wave me back. Utter gall! It really burned me so I decided to go give him back exactly what I had gotten. I stomped down the stairs and headed right toward him, anticipating my retort. When I got to his side, he surprised the heck out of me when, with a rose in his hand, he bent down on one knee and asked me to dance! Can you believe it? Smart guy. Suave, charming . . . warning bells

4

went off in my head. *Danger. Caution. Careful.*

I fell in love that night. Something hit me like a thunderbolt. No question about it. We spent the evening together, in a booth that is, exchanging vital statistics. We started out drinking Miller Lites (we liked the same beer) then we switched to Martinis, dry, two olives please. I couldn't believe it when the lights came on, it was 2:00 a.m., last call. His name was Elias. It took me awhile to pronounce it. I'd never heard the name before. He was Cuban. Handsome, funny, intelligent. There was such a connection. It was something like: I feel like I *know you.*

My friends were yelling for me to leave with them. His friend, Don, gave him the "thumbs up" sign and left. The party was over, it was time to leave. I bid my friends goodbye at the door and let doe-eyes walk me to my car. He got into the passenger's side and we sat and talked some more. I already knew that he didn't have any children, and was separated from his wife but I also noticed that he wore a wedding band on his right hand. A Spanish tradition. What did that mean . . . separated, but not divorced? Still wearing the wedding band? I'm Italian. In my family, if you're married, you wear the ring. Period. On the left hand. I let it ride. I liked him too much not to let it ride. I told him I was divorced and had two kids. I didn't want to

5

get married again. I owned my own home in Coral Springs, Florida, a nice, relatively safe, family-oriented community. I was the manager of a marketing communications department for a major computer manu-facturer. I had been with the same company for 10 years and I had my life planned. When my kids were grown and gone . . . I was moving to my condo on Hollywood beach. The only thing I needed was a "wife" to take care of all the things I barely had time to take care of. He laughed. I loved his laugh.

He had given me his business card but I wouldn't give him mine. No phone numbers. No way. You never know. I'll call you. He mentioned that maybe I'd like to go to some charity function with him on Friday night.

"Ah, yeah, sure, I'll call you." I had a hard time believing that he was involved in any charity function. I didn't trust him at all so of course I didn't believe him. I don't trust easily. But, he made me feel GREAT. I was on cloud nine talking to him. I loved his voice, his hair, and that gorgeous mouth. His beautiful eyes. He gave me butterflies.

It was time to go home. Get out of my car. He leaned over and kissed me and I thought I'd die. My heart was beating in my mouth! What the heck was happening to me? It was obviously love. I never expected to fall in love so fast. But, when you find the right person . . . it all becomes so clear!

He got out of the car and came around to my side, leaned in and asked: "Do you wanna do a hot tub?" I couldn't believe it. Get lost. No way. Good night. See ya!

Of course I daydreamed about him the entire next day at work. I kept his business card on my desk . . . said his name over and over and smiled alot. On Friday I called him. We agreed that I might be bored at his charity function so instead decided to meet for cocktails later that evening. I coerced a girlfriend, who just happened to be a cop, into coming with me to meet him. We had our "codes" defined if I wanted her to leave me there or stay and drive me back home. You never know! I also figured that if he didn't show up (my insecurities!) at least she and I could have a good time. He showed. On time. Looking great. He had that Don Johnson, Miami Vice look and my girlfriend said . . . "That's him? Damn, did you luck out!" I smiled and thought *we'll see*!

I brought him a jar of green olives in honor of our previous "Martini" night. He brought me a flashlight from his charity function! Yes . . . a flashlight. I still have it. I thought it was cute. I thought everything about him was cute. My friend left. We danced, talked and

7

drank. It was a memorable evening. First dates always are. We just couldn't seem to get enough of each other.

So, we dated. We would see each other on Wednesday and Friday nights during that first month. We'd meet on the beach on Saturday mornings and spend the day together. If we couldn't do that then we would definitely see each other on Sundays. We talked for hours and hours, totally consumed with each other. We probably would have spent every waking moment together but we had jobs and I had two kids that needed me.

The high didn't last too long. One Saturday morning he came to pick me up and he looked so sad. We went to a local park and sat on a bench and he broke my heart for the first time. They were reconciling…trying to work things out. I was devastated. That was that . . . it was over. Goodbye. Good luck.

I wanted to forget him; I didn't want to be depressed. But, I felt sick to my stomach and very empty. It was an awful feeling. My friends consoled me. For two weeks I felt sorry for myself but then I resumed dating a pilot I had met long before Eli.

After a month of moping around, all my resolutions to forget him went out the window when I decided to call *him*. Just to say, "hi, how are you?" We met for drinks and we started to see each other

8

again. But it was different this time. He was *married* for gosh sakes! We couldn't spend the holidays together. We couldn't go to functions together. We couldn't even go to local festivals together. He was afraid someone he knew would see us. It was awful. I had feelings for him that I never had for anyone else. But, I also felt like "the other woman." Being with him constantly compromised my morals and went against everything I was teaching my kids. It wasn't right. And, yet, we continued.

For the next seven months, we were on again and off again. It was a wonderful time and yet a time so filled with guilt and feelings of betrayal . . . on both our parts. Yet we couldn't seem to stop seeing each other. Once, when the kids were visiting with their dad, we took the day off from work, met at 6:00 a.m. and drove south to the Keys. We had a blast. It was one for the scrapbooks. (I saved everything, as a token of our love, and put my "stuff" in a scrapbook.) We danced in the moonlight on the beach, fed each other jumbo shrimp, and of course, drank our giddy heads off. But, it was always over too soon. And, I always wanted more.

We stopped "seeing each other" seven times in seven months. I just couldn't handle it and there were times when he just couldn't handle me. I didn't make demands on him; I just had a hard time justifying being with "a married man." When he said he had to go home . . . I would cringe. When he couldn't accompany me to a social or business affair, I would get angry, not with him, at myself. I had little understanding, and yet I understood.

One of us would always weaken and call the other. Or, on a couple of occasions, we ran into each other at Cadillac Jacks. When I went there, I would either pray that he wasn't there (he should be at home with his wife!) or I prayed that he would be there. It was crazy!

Finally, I decided that enough was really enough. I was a wreck. I cried too much. My kids knew that something wasn't right with their mom and they started to resent Eli. We met one gorgeous Saturday morning at our usual spot on Hollywood beach and I told him that I just couldn't do it anymore. It was too painful to be with him. I told him to please go home to his wife and make an honest attempt at reconciliation. I begged him not to call me unless . . .! I promised that I would never call him again and wished him nothing but happiness. It was honestly the saddest day of my life. I watched him walk off the beach and I stayed and cried until there was nothing left inside of me. I went home and vowed to move on . . . for my sake as well as my kids' sake. I packed all the "stuff" he had ever given me, along with the photos I had of him, into a large box marked: DO NOT OPEN. I

10

hid the box in my garage and told myself: THAT IS IT! OVER. CAPUT.

I didn't hear from him. I didn't call him. I stayed away from Cadillac Jacks, just in case. I went back with the pilot. Boring, but single. Safe.

I walked around with a "pretend I'm happy" face and went about my life. It wasn't the same without him in it. I didn't want the kids to see how unhappy I was so I went out on weekends, entertained friends at home, went to work like a good Mom, spent time with the kids when they wanted to see me and generally led a normal, single mom's life.

At 7:30 a.m. on Saturday, July 9, I was heading out the door to catch the early sun on the beach before I had to take care of my Saturday errands when the phone rang. I figured it was for my daughter, Shannon, and I was going to let it ring and wake her up. I changed my mind at the last moment and grabbed it. It was *him.* My heart started racing uncontrollably, I broke out in a sweat and my stomach was doing flip-flops.

"Hi . . . what's going on? How are you?" *You're not supposed to be calling me.*

"Can you meet me on the beach? I have something I need to talk to

11

you about," he said.

I had stopped going to "our beach." I found a new "my" beach, but, of course, I agreed to meet him. It must be important. We hadn't seen each other or spoken in six weeks. Given our short history that was truly a long time for us.

"Yes, I'll be there in half an hour; is everything Okay?" "Uh . . . yeah. Just come down to the beach."

I was scared but I didn't know what I was scared about. I just knew he was going to tell me that his wife was pregnant. But, why would he call *me* to tell me that? Who knows? My mind wasn't working right. I immediately called Beverly, a supportive friend and believer in true love, and told her. She said GO! I went.

"Hi."

"Hi. What's going on? What's so important that I had to meet you here?"

"It's over. We're getting divorced. It's not meant to be. I tried. It was over a long time ago. I just had to be sure. I don't feel anything anymore. I'm in love with you." What could I do? What could I say? I just kissed him...hard, long.

You could almost say, "the rest is history," but not quite. His divorce was final in August. I wanted him to move in with me. He was emphatic about NOT living with me.

His mom and dad are very traditional and needed time to adjust to his divorce. The last thing he wanted to do was spring ME on them. *Mom and Dad, I'd like you to meet Deb, she's divorced with two kids, but has a great job and has her act together, and I'm in love with her.* Yeah, sure. But, I did meet them one day when his dad was in the hospital. The hospital, of all places. We went to visit him. They didn't make any comments about me being with him but I knew they were concerned. We stayed low-key. But, we were finally able to go "out in public" together. It validated our relationship. I wanted to go everywhere with him. Be seen everywhere . . . together. He introduced me to Cuban food; I cooked Italian food for him. We gave each other silly cards and little gifts that only the two of us could understand. We started to finish each other's sentences, read each other's glances and knew by a tone of voice whether each other's mood was good or bad. We met each other's friends and relatives and attended social functions together. We were a couple.

He made himself available for my kids. He had the patience to deal with two teenagers and the wisdom to know when to leave the room so that I could deal with them. He didn't try to "be their father," he didn't impose himself on them. He was just there when they

13

seemed to need it and in the long run, this strategy worked perfectly for us.

We *talked* about getting married. I couldn't believe I was even talking about getting married. Marriage had been the furthest thing from my mind, before Eli. Impossible. We talked about how we would have to combine all our belongings, all our "stuff." And boy did we have "stuff." I had a house. He had a townhouse. I had a car. He had a car *plus* a company car. How did we get from yours and mine to "ours?" And, then we had to consider my kids. Especially Shannon. She was a senior in high school at the time. She wasn't thrilled that I was even seeing him again. We agreed that we wouldn't do anything until Shannon was out of high school, and that was about a year or so away. No sense in upsetting *that* apple cart! More than once I asked him to move in with me. It made perfect sense to me. We were always together anyway. But, he wouldn't do it. He just didn't believe in "living together." I, on the other hand, was scared to death of getting married and would have preferred to try our arrangement out ahead of time. I couldn't budge his decision! I learned how stubborn he could be.

We *talked* about having children. When we first met, I had made it perfectly clear to him that I had no intentions of having any

14

more kids. I was done. I had my tubes tied when my son was three years old. He told me he didn't care if he had kids or not. It wasn't a big deal to him. I tried to believe him but I found myself working through thoughts like: *every man wants an image of himself; every man wants a son to carry on his name; I can't deprive him of never having children and experiencing that kind of unrequited love.* He convinced me that we would live a different kind of lifestyle . . . one filled with traveling and romantic evenings, just the two of us. We moved on.

On October 21, 1988, one week before our "one year of having met" anniversary, Eli wanted to introduce me to the Seybold Building in Miami. The Seybold Building turned out to be literally floors and floor of jewelers. I had never seen so much gold and diamonds in one place before. They should have had armored guards standing at the doorways. It's a fabulous place. (When he mentions going to The Seybold Building now . . . I'm ready to go before he finishes the sentence!) We drove down to Miami with one goal in mind: to buy an ankle bracelet for me to mark our one-year anniversary.

Eli had lived in Miami since he was 15 years old so he knew Dade county inside and out. At this time, I had lived in Florida, Broward county to be exact, for 16 years and rarely ventured over the

15

county lines so driving into Miami was an adventure for me. Miami is a world all in its own!

We got to The Seybold Building and I felt like I'd died and gone to gold heaven. Everywhere I turned, I saw more gold, diamonds, rubies, sapphires and all kinds of precious stones. I didn't really think I would be able to make a decision about a bracelet. Just let me look for awhile . . . please. I dragged Eli up and down hallways, in and out of stores and finally stopped in a store called Freddy's where I began browsing at the different bracelets. I was trying on a few little trinkets when Eli asked me which diamond shape I liked the most. "Marquis," I said.

He called me over to a long counter and Freddy himself came out with a tray full of gorgeous, sparkling, cut diamonds. Still, I didn't think too much of it until Freddy started choosing various diamonds and putting them into different settings for me to approve or disapprove. I was having a great time. This was an extraordinary way to spend a Saturday afternoon! After viewing four or five different settings, I finally fell in love with a gorgeous marquis in a single gold setting. The perfect solitaire. It just beckoned me. Freddy said to Eli: "Do you want me to mount it so you can give it to her?"
Eli replied, "Heck, I haven't even asked her to marry me yet."

I was absolutely stunned. My mouth went dry and I was speechless until Eli started clapping his hands to get the attention of all the customers in the store. I was laughing so hard, barely able to speak but I kept telling him: "No, no . . . don't do it here . . . NO . . . this is too embarrassing."

It didn't stop him. He made sure all the customers were watching and then went down on one knee and asked me to marry him right there in the store. What could I say? Between the laughter and the tears, I said yes to the bursting sound of applause. I walked out with the marquis and my fiancée. It wasn't planned that way, it just happened. And that is sort of the way our life has been.

I've always believed in fate. What's meant to be will happen. And I've always trusted my gut instincts. If it feels right . . . it must be. Eli had the same philosophies as I did. We both just knew when something was right! It's an inner sense that guides you along life's path.

However, I still hadn't reconciled my feelings about Eli not experiencing the joys of parenthood. After we got engaged, my thoughts and feelings on the subject were even more intense. I wanted to build a home together, have a family together . . . the old "nesting" bug hit and hit me hard. I was (and still am!) so in love with him. I wanted to

17

have his baby. It was an all-consuming feeling of the need to share a child together . . . our child. Our creation. We talked until we exhausted the subject and I finally made an appointment with my gynecologist to try to get answers to some tough questions.

I was 34 years old the day I asked my OB/GYN if my tubal ligation could be reversed. He reviewed the records of the procedure that had occurred many years prior and assured me that, according to the notes in my record, I would be able to have the operation reversed and hopefully get pregnant again. My gynecologist referred me to a fertility center and to the team of Dr. Wayne and Dr. David. He said these doctors could further judge my condition and perform the surgery.

I was ecstatic. My cheeks hurt from smiling so much. I could have a baby *after all*. Eli's baby! On the drive home, I thought about the day I had made the decision to have my tubes tied. The doctor tried to talk me out of it because I was only 22 years old. NO WAY. I was so determined to get it taken care of. I didn't want any more kids. Never in my life would I have dreamed that I would want to reverse such a decision.

Eli was waiting for me at my house when I came home and he could tell by the smile crinkles that we were two very lucky people.

Standing in the foyer of my home, I wrapped my arms around his neck and very quietly, with tears in my eyes, told him, "We can have a baby." It was like someone had given us the greatest gift on earth!

Little did we know that just wanting to have a baby would take us down a five-year road filled with dips, curves, hills and very rocky mountains. Nothing is ever easy in life and you can never take anything for granted! Although we both already knew and lived by this philosophy, we didn't know how much we would really wind up believing in it.

He Said...

My life was just in a wee bit of disarray. After being on the executive fast track for the previous three years, I had suffered some hard times of late. I had recently weathered a bad computer billing conversion at work, a new phone system that failed to work, and a few other snafus that I was taking the brunt of. My marriage was headed in the wrong direction, and physically I wasn't feeling all that great for a 28-year old. Wednesday nights my buddy Don and I would escape the real world for a few hours and park ourselves like statues at the south counter of this local hangout called *Cadillac Jacks*.

Don and I would start the night with an exchange of healthy

corporate conversation, solve all of the company's ills by declaring that we both were ready to become Vice Presidents. We then would proceed to reorganize the division by moving all the players around. After one beer and five minutes of that, we would graduate to matters of more global consequence, like the length of a particular skirt, or the combined mass weight of all the breasts in the room.

Don was definitely there to meet someone although his criteria for suitable companionship was stricter than a barracks check by a platoon sergeant. I was there because I did not want to be at home, but by the same token, there was this piece of paper that said I wasn't a free man. My attitude was, I'm here to have a few beers, watch the crowd, have a few laughs and go home. No agenda, no mission.

And so every Wednesday we would replay this scenario, and over time we began to be part of the crowd of regulars, sort of a free membership to the *"Looking for Love in All the Wrong Places"* club.

On this particular October night we arrived on time, as usual and grabbed a couple of beers and headed for our spot. Twenty minutes into one of our heated conversations, I noticed out of my left peripheral vision a woman coming my way, and as I was turning she reached the counter, smiled and in one hurried breath said "Hi, wanna dance?" A million thoughts were racing through my mind at that particular moment. *No, I don't wanna dance, can't you see I'm in the middle of this important conversation? Don't you see that I still have half a beer left? Don't you realize that I'M not here to dance, but rather to purge myself from all the things that trouble me at this point in my life?*

But as all those rude replies raced through my mind in that split second, I was able to gracefully decline without a trace of insult, or a clue as to the inner status of my psyche.

"No thanks, I don't really care for this song, maybe later, I'll come look for you," and picked up my beer and took another swig. She smiled and mumbled something about getting down on one knee and begging her later, but I wasn't really focusing on her response. Don was already lecturing me about the perils of turning females down when they ask you to dance.

"Don, PUT A CORK IN IT AND BUY ME ANOTHER MILLER LIGHT," I retorted as I lit another Benson & Hedges.

The evening continued as usual, music, beers, laughter, but fate had it that this evening would be different. About an hour after the exchange with the "wanna dance lady," I decided to return the offer. I made my way up to the platform where she was hanging out and walked up to her ready, positioned and customarily cocky. (Deb swears

I was waving for her to come down to where I was standing; I don't re-call it the same way!) "Okay," I said with full confidence, and appar-ent arrogance, "would you like to dance to this song?"

As her eyes widened not with jubilation because I was asking her to dance, but with the opportunity to even the score, my legs began to mysteriously buckle into halves as if some unknown, uncontrollable force was directing them. Before I knew what had happened I was on my knee begging for another chance. I do not remember who was more surprised at my actions, this stranger I was compromising my machismo to, or the macho himself.

Somehow, as the evening progressed, it didn't seem to mat-ter. The first dance led to hours of conversation, half a dozen Miller Lights, a few potent martinis, several more dances, and yet more conversation. I blinked my eyes and the house was reminding all the patrons about last call. Geez it was 2:00 a.m., where did the night go? Where did Don go? Oh yeah, I remember. Sometime around midnight my buddy exited, and from afar he gave me that *"tell me about it in the morning, hope you get lucky"* wink.

Several times during the conversation I noticed that repeated attempts at giving this interesting woman my business card had failed which must have meant that she probably was not interested.

Nevertheless as we collected our things and headed for the parking lot, a million thoughts were racing through my mind.

We sat in her car for awhile and talked some more. I consider myself a people person and people persons talk alot so this was normal. What wasn't normal was that Debbie was a people person too but her conversation had substance, and it was of much interest to me. This was not the typical bar encounter. Usually the people I met in bars were hollow, shallow, phony, but not this time. This "chick" was cool.

Well as the moment of truth approached I had to decide how I was going to close the evening so in typical male fashion I relied on the approach that came most natural.

"So do you want to go do a hot tub?"

After several seconds of silence, followed by a big smile and mutual laughter, she very politely told me to "hit the road." What was great about the rejection was that the little voice inside of me said *You lucked out bub, 'cause she didn't get mad.* This was good because I really did want to see her again. God, we had so much to still talk about. So I told her that I understood and I said that I hoped she understood that I had to ask and she again politely smiled and brushed it off. I finally told her about a function I was working later that week and that I would love for her to come to it if she liked. I leaned over and kissed her goodnight and left.

Later that week I was in my office one morning going through my corporate routines when the phone rang. It was *her*, I recognized her voice immediately. I have to admit I was surprised she called because I didn't think she had picked up my business card from the table, and because I really didn't think she was all that interested. I mean statistically how many of us really call when we say we're going to call? Well after some chitchat we decided that she probably would not enjoy the function I was working Friday night so we agreed to meet afterwards at a club in Ft Lauderdale.

Friday night I was doing my thing at this charity function with and for Don, since he was president of the local chapter. Around 9:00 p.m., I asked Don if I could split to pursue this emotional endeavor without hurting his function? I guess he must have seen the adrenaline in my eyes, so without any hesitation he said, "Go get 'em tiger!" Ah, now I understood. Don saw hormones not adrenaline. Well whatever Don thought he saw was fine with me, I just wanted to go. Thirty minutes later I was walking into this club looking for Debbie and I found her sitting at the bar with another gal.

"Hiiiii" radiated from that terrific smile as I approached. Later that evening I learned that her friend was a cop, and I thought, I must look like some nut if she feels she needs to bring a cop. I had learned something about this woman with the unexplainable magnetism. Despite her open approach to living life to the fullest, there was a cautious and calculating streak in her, a quality I would eventually admire.

The next seven months were the best and worst in my life. As I continued to see Debbie I was still wrestling with the fixed components of my life. I was still married but not really living a married life. My wife and I were together, then apart. Patching up our differences one day, filing for divorce the next. I was on a marital roller coaster, which was aggravated by the fact that I was on a romantic roller coaster with Debbie. Anyone that tells you that "the other woman" will understand doesn't understand themselves.

Eventually Debbie and I fell into a pattern. We would spend three terrific hours together, then snap back into reality, fight about the fact that I wasn't a free man, and part mad at each other, only to do it over and over and over again.

At one point I actually had an "I don't give a damn" attitude. I wanted out of my marriage but couldn't get past the guilt, so I figured that my wife would eventually learn about my indiscretions and drop me like a hot potato. On the other hand I rationalized that I had always been candid with Debbie about my status, so I wasn't going to sweat it anymore with her either.

One day on the beach it all came to a head, and Debbie and I agreed that we could not continue on this path of destruction. For every moment of pleasure we gave each other, we passed on hours of torture, and too many people were at risk of being hurt.

So she told me we were done and I was actually relieved because I always knew deep down that I could not and would not resolve my situation at home with this relationship clouding the picture. I had to fix or abandon my four-year investment based on the merits or failures of the marriage only, with no distractions, alibi's, or third party influences. I remember walking away from Deb that day on the beach, relieved of this enormous burden on one hand, and feeling like I had a dagger twisting in my stomach on the other. I kept telling myself that I was doing the right thing, and that eventually the dagger would be absorbed in the system through the emotional digestive process.

By July of that year I had come to terms with my marriage, and with clean conscience had made my decision to move on with my life. My ex-wife was and is a lovely human being, the type of woman that men would kill for, but not the person planted on this earth to be my soul mate, and I certainly was not the man that was going to make her happy. So in typical Eli fashion, once the decision gets made, the wheels start moving and there is no hesitation and no turning back. I had turned a critical corner in my life.

One Saturday morning I went into the office and started making telephone calls to the people that mattered in my life to tell them about the decision I had made. Eventually I built up enough courage to dial Debbie's number, worried that she would hang up on me when she heard my voice for fear of opening the wounds up again. To my surprise she recognized my voice immediately, didn't hang up on me, and to my real amazement, agreed to see me that morning at my request. No questions, no conditions, and most importantly to me in retrospect, no hesitation.

By noon that day I had brought Deb up to date on my life, and purged myself of all my inner true feelings for her. I wanted us to have a real shot now without the cloud. Let's find out if we are really good together. Her smile, her laugh, her tears, her kiss, her touch . . . they all said Yes, Yes, Yes!

The next several months were great. I was learning how to be the real me again. Laughing, experimenting, squeezing the juice out of life every day. Some people were convinced I was suffering from *Terminal Rebound,* others supported my apparent direction. My parents, who are traditional and somewhat conservative, were still dealing with my recent breakup, and were not prepared for that Saturday night phone call. " Hey guys guess what? I just got engaged!"

The next several weeks were spent planning the "big day," and trying to convince my family that I was not doing drugs or under any special evil love potion. After all, this lady was divorced, she had two grown kids, and she was older than their first born offspring. By Thanksgiving the excrement had hit the fan, and hit it good. My parents, whom I loved very much, and my fiancé, whom I loved very much, had me between a rock and a hard place.

In the former days I would have resolved the situation by picking sides, and giving the other side an ultimatum. But I had done a certain amount of maturing in recent times, and I was determined to have my cake and eat it too. By Christmas both sides actually sat down to dinner together, and hence another dimension of this new lifestyle seemed to be under control.

I remember thinking about what Deb's kids must have thought when they learned the true story about our rocky seven-month court-ship. As our "till death do us part" date approached, my relationship with the kids started to focus clearer. Buddy, at 13, decided I was somewhat cool and tolerable. Shannon, at 16, quickly approaching the wise age of 17, had pretty much made up her mind that I was the "cheats on his wife" type, and found me to be one big threat.

Quite clearly, this dimension was not only going to require diligent effort, but was going to take time. Oh well. They were part of the package, the package that so many people warned me about, but I was not phased. I knew that I was a pretty cool human being, fair, honest, warm and caring. Bottom line: they were either going to like me or hate me for me, because ME is who I'M going to be.

One afternoon I sat them both down and told them just that. Everyone knew the jury was out, so we decided to do the rational thing . . . move on.

Having a baby soon became part of the master plan. I knew well in advance of "Will you marry me?" that Deb had her tubes tied after her son was born, and that having a baby was going to be more than a bottle of wine in front of a fireplace on a passionate night. Steps had to be taken, questions had to be asked, and in the realm of all the good things that were happening to me in my life I just figured that it would all work out when the time came. As a matter of fact, after a consultation with her gynecologist, who had a copy of her records, Deb came home one afternoon and said "Sweetheart good news . . . the doctor says the process can be reversed. We can have a baby!" Another piece of the puzzle was fitting right into place, easy as pie . . . or so I thought.

Chapter Two

The Engagement, Wedding & Newlywed Days

She Said...

We were walking on air after we got engaged and then found out there was a possibility of having a baby. Talk about two happy people! We wanted to share our good news with everyone . . . immediately.

With that diamond sparkling on my left hand, we headed to "our" place, Cadillac Jacks, to see if any of our friends were there. We were just bursting with our news. We walked the entire place and found absolutely no one. Of course not. It was Saturday night . . . date night. Oh well. We went home. Even the kids weren't there. I tried calling a few of my girlfriends but no one was home. We had to wait until the next day to spring our news on anyone.

That night we considered the reactions we'd get from the people we loved. This could get difficult. After all, it was only a few months since his divorce was final and here he was getting married again. What would people say? What would people think? We cared, yet it was really our life to live . . . although we didn't want to cause stress for anyone else. The reactions, from my kids (my parents both died in 1987) and Eli's parents, were predictable. With the exception of a few very good friends, no one really said very much. Everyone had skeptical faces and dire predictions. We talked until we were blue in the face, trying to explain, but in the end we had to do what was best for us. And we figured eventually they would all understand and be able to see and feel our love for one another.

The kids were concerned about themselves and moving out of our home. They didn't want to leave their friends, their schools, and their lives! To put it mildly, Eli's family thought we were being too impulsive. We assured the kids that we weren't going anywhere until Shannon had graduated from high school, but after that we couldn't guarantee anything. His family eventually accepted his decision to remarry and gave him the love and support he wanted.

One day in November we found ourselves in the mall with the kids . . . trying to decide a wedding date. We all wrote dates on the back of napkins, folded them up and put them into Buddy's hat and I picked the date out of the hat! March 18, 1989 would be the beginning of a new journey for all of us.

We began making wedding plans. Eli was a very active partici-pant in just about every issue. We decided to keep it very small. No more than 50 people and we would have the ceremony on the patio at my home. We wanted our family to somehow be part of the ceremony so we asked both kids (Shannon was 16 at the time and Buddy was al-most 14) to participate as well as his parents. Eli's sister, Marilyn, was a notary so we asked her to perform the ceremony for us. We wrote our own wedding invitation and our wedding vows. We contacted caterers and bought new outfits; ordered a wedding cake (chocolate, of course), asked friends to take video and photography for us and met with a florist. We decided to have a Saturday midmorning brunch with champagne and mimosas, croissants and crepes. After the wedding and reception, we would take off for a week's cruise to the Caribbean. My maid of honor and good friend, Beverly, offered to stay at the house to be with the kids. It was all set.

The morning dawned gloriously . . . bright sunshine and a

33

gorgeous blue sky. I woke up on cloud nine. And one look at Eli told me that he was right up there with me. It went off with few problems. Everyone knew their parts. We rehearsed the night before and everything seemed in order. We giggled when we saw the video of the kids walking down the "aisle" . . . Buddy didn't offer his arm and Shannon didn't take it. They both looked scared stiff. The music for my processional was too long and we waited up at the "altar" for a good five minutes for it to end. We laughed.

We gave each of our family members a corsage as a symbol of uniting the two families. Eli's best man, Wayne, delivered a flawless, loving toast for happiness, and, we drank whatever anyone handed us, mingled among our guests, danced when we were supposed to, and threw the bouquet and garter. We cut the cake and didn't give in to the temptation to smash it into each other's faces. We finally felt like the genuine love and happiness of our friends surrounded us. It was beautiful. And it was over before we knew it. It seemed like the whole thing was a big dream . . . a dream that came true! We hardly remembered the ride to the port to go on the cruise. It was truly euphoric . . . a natural high.

When we returned from an absolutely wonderful honeymoon, we watched our video at least 100 times and saw people that we didn't even know were there! And we found 50 bottles of champagne in our bar. When we set up the bar the night before, we didn't put all the champagne out because we wanted it to be chilled. We totally forgot about it in the morning.

It was good to be home and to start settling down into married life . . . again! Eli moved in. We didn't fight about closet space or privacy, just the lack of both. Eli had alot of adjustments to make; he took on a ready-made package . . . with lots of history. Everyone had adjustments to make and everyone made mistakes in judgment.

Buddy adapted easily. He's the charmer of the family with an easy going personality. "Sure, that's okay with me." Shannon, on the other hand, didn't want Eli intruding in our lives and was afraid that I wouldn't be *available* for her anymore. She adapted slowly.

We didn't mention to anyone that we wanted to have a baby yet. We were still letting them adjust to us being married. But, we did plan to move forward with our desire to get rid of "his" and "hers" and get to "ours."

First on our agenda was to find a way to get down to just one car. My car was a couple of years old, but Eli had a new car (only six months old), plus the company car. We debated keeping his "new" car and selling my "old" car but we decided to see if we couldn't just dump both cars and buy a new "our" car. Off we went to the dealerships. We told our "two for one trade" story to five dealerships before we found one that would do business with us. Most of them thought we were nuts. Who cared? We had our goal in mind . . . and our minds made up. We traded both cars in for a brand spanking new black Grand Prix. Boy, did we take a bath.

Since we each had a house-full of "stuff," we needed options for furniture consolidation. I wanted to keep most of mine since it was practically new, except for my bedroom set. I didn't want any of his. We practically gave all his furniture and kitchen necessities away to his secretary. She was thrilled to have designer furniture at such bargain basement prices. But, you've got to do what you've got to do in order to obtain your goals. And, we were doing it. Eli's townhouse was smaller than my house and we weren't sure everything was even going to fit into it if we wound up moving there. Oh well, we'd deal with that one later. We decided to keep all my furniture except for my bedroom suite, and we kept all of our electronics, including a television for every room!

Shannon graduated from high school in June and we put both my house and the townhouse up for sale. My house sold first. I was glad and sad at the same time. I loved living there and I had gotten attached to the house. But, it was time to move on.

My son, who would be starting high school soon, decided it was time for a change for him too. One morning, out of the blue, he told me that he wanted to go live with his dad and attend high school in Lakeland, FL. *Where the heck did that come from?* After much discussion with his father, I cut the strings and let him explore a new life.

Amidst sadness and tears, for my son's departure and our moving out of the house, and out of Coral Springs, we packed the house and moved to Eli's townhouse. Shannon reluctantly moved with us. The townhouse was smaller than our house, and Shannon and I hated the neighborhood. Nobody, including Eli, liked living there. In the long run, it was a blessing that Buddy moved to his dad's since the three of us were constantly on top of each other. Shannon began packing a bag and spending weekends back in Coral Springs with her best friend, Monique. But, Eli and I were optimistic that the place would sell quickly and so we started to look for "our" dream house. We explored all types of homes in Dade and Broward County for the next six months, but didn't see anything that really hit us.

The broker assured us that we would have no problem selling the townhouse but after six months, he hadn't shown the place once! We knew we weren't overpriced and the place was in great shape. The problem was that there were just too many townhouses on the market. The meaning of the term "a buyer's market" was quickly apparent. We were glad that we hadn't found a house that we loved yet since we were stuck with the dinosaur.

In the meantime, we decided to make an appointment with the fertility doctors that my gynecologist had recommended. We wanted to talk about a reverse tubal ligation.

Our first meeting with Dr. David was basically a "fill out all the paperwork" and "let's talk a little about your private life." We dutifully filled in the blanks on what seemed to be an absurd amount of paperwork. Both of us were quite nervous, yet excited, as we waited patiently in the small office to talk to the doctor that hopefully would reverse my long-ago decision so we could add to the family.

Dr. David walked in the room and for some unknown reason, him and Eli just did not click. I liked him immediately. And later when I met his partner, Dr. Wayne, I liked him just as well. I could work with either of them and since it was *my body* that was going to be probed and poked at, I figured my husband didn't need to be best friends with my doctors.

Dr. David asked a series of questions about our lifestyle, habits and routines. It was pretty tense in the office until he asked us how often we had sex. I turned beet red and just looked at Eli. My husband, in usual Eli humor, answered the doctor with a question: "Who are you asking, me or her?" To which Dr. David replied: "What's that supposed to mean?" That broke the ice and we all started to laugh. At the end of the session, we were told that the good doctor would have to perform a laparoscopy in order to determine the condition of my tubes. In other words, once he looked inside, he'd be able to tell whether he could reattach the tubes. We scheduled the surgery to be done as soon as possible.

I was scared to death. I hate needles and IV's. And there I was, lying on a rollaway hospital bed, naked under a hospital gown and white sheet, teeth chattering, with a needle in my hand. Eli kept making wise cracks to make me laugh but I didn't see anything funny about this procedure. They wheeled me into the surgical area where I saw Dr. David waiting for me. I was glad to see him and somewhat reassured. The next thing I knew, I was waking up in the recovery room.

Dr. David was standing next to me and when I was fully awake, he gently broke the heart wrenching news to me. "I'm sorry Deb, but I'm not going to be able to reverse this tubal because your tubes were cut too far down and there's very little left to reattach." He also told me that he had taken care of some endometriosis spots and that I shouldn't worry about anything else. Yeah, sure! I had just been told that I couldn't have a child because I didn't have any workable fallopian tubes and I wasn't supposed to worry about it! I immediately started crying and asking for my husband. Dr. David patted me on the shoulder, and tried his best to comfort me by telling me that there were other options and to make an appointment to see him the following week. He left me alone with my tears and the awful thoughts of having to tell my husband that he wouldn't be able to have any kids. At least not with me!

After 15 minutes or so, Dr. David came back into the recovery room and still found me alone and crying. He got pretty mad at one of the nurses and started to yell at her: "Hasn't anyone gone to get her husband in here yet?" Eli appeared moments later, worried, haggard and upset. He already knew. He held me while I cried and I told him how awfully sorry I was. I blamed myself for a flippant decision I had made so many years ago.

We met with Dr. David the following week and he showed us the video they had made of the results of the laparoscopy. It was pretty obvious that I had very little fallopian tubes left. He wanted to talk to us about adoption and about a procedure called *In Vitro Fertilization, IVF*, but we were too emotionally drained to talk about anything else that day and decided that we would schedule another appointment in the near future. We took all the literature he gave us and left.

It wasn't long after that visit to Dr. David that we suffered another blow. This one was one of immediate concern for me. The computer company I worked for was bought out by another firm and I got laid-off. It was devastating. I'd worked there for more than ten years. I started as a secretary and worked my way up to a marketing management position. I "grew up" there. I worked hard for what I had accomplished. I couldn't believe I had to *look for a job*. The only consolation was that I wasn't the only one. So many people were getting pink slips that the television crews were on campus to try to capture a few parting remarks. I believe that everything happens for a reason and even though I didn't know what the reason was then, I knew there had to be a correlation in the future.

Eli had his own work problems. He had just moved into a new position as a Service Manager for the gas company. Alien territory for him. He had his plate full with new problems of managing 60+ employees. And, he still had to deal with a stepdaughter that thought the world had ended because we moved from Coral Springs. The last thing he needed was an unemployed wife. I felt guilty, defensive, angry, and depressed all at the same time. Geez, what a way to start out a

41

marriage. We would really be lucky if we made it through this first year. Good thing I could cook!

I updated my resume and started looking for a new job. I collected unemployment, something I had never done before. It wasn't easy finding a job and I was getting bored with being at home. It wasn't fair that Eli was the only breadwinner. I should be pulling my weight too. So I decided that unemployment compensation just wasn't going to cut it and I could make more money working at ANY job. My bruised ego and self-esteem would be smoothed if I were just doing something. It was October when I applied to Macy's to be a jewelry sales clerk for the Christmas season. What the heck. It was better than nothing, better than being on unemployment and at least I had something to do every day. I found out that I was a pretty good sales person and I loved being in contact with so many people everyday. I continued my hunt for a "professional" job and went on a few interviews but nothing was happening. Finally, one day in early December, I got a call from the Human Resources Manager at a healthcare company in Miami. I had sent my resume in response to a Senior Marketing Communications Specialist advertisement I saw in the Sunday paper. She wanted to know if I was still interested. YES! Most definitely. Sign me up . . . or where do I sign?!

I interviewed with the Human Resources representative and then with the Director of Marketing Communications. It sounded like the job was made for me, and I loved the idea of working for a big company again. I got the standard, "We'll make our decision in a week," line and left feeling pretty good about it. I didn't hear from them again until three weeks later. By then I had resolved that my instincts had failed me and that I had read the signals wrong. Oh well, move on.

But when they called again, I was elated. They wanted me to come back for a second interview. I gladly complied. This time I talked with the Director again and then with the Vice President of Marketing. I liked the company even more and the job sounded even better. The interviews went well and I left feeling as though it would be only a matter of days before I had an offer letter in my hands. WRONG!

Christmas came and went before I finally heard from the Director. "We're working out some internal problems, we really want you to start here soon. Please bear with us and we'll be calling you very shortly." I thought this was pretty unconventional, to have the Director calling me pretty much saying that I had the job, just hang in there. Well, nothing else was cooking so what did I have to lose? He called me again a few weeks later to deliver the same type of message. "Yes,

yes, I'm still interested, but when is this going to happen?" "Soon," was all he could say.

Around the end of January, Macy's offered me a permanent position. The Christmas rush was over and they were laying off the temporary help but were keeping those people who had achieved high sales records. I was flattered, but really not interested in making Macy's my permanent career. However, I did like the discounts I got for working there! I bought quite a few suits, in anticipation of going back to work for a "real" company! I told them I needed a few days to think it over and was able to stall for two weeks when finally, the offer call came in from the healthcare company. YES, YES, I accept.

I started working for my new company in mid-February, 1990. In 1991, I was promoted to Manager of Marketing Communications and I was loving every minute of it. This company offered an entire smorgasbord of benefits. Now I knew why I had been laid-off from my computer company. My health insurance covered IVF, the computer company did not and neither did the gas company. *Everything happens for a reason!*

Maybe it was time to consider the other baby options that Dr. David had suggested . . . the IVF option. We made another appointment with Dr. David to talk about the IVF program. What the heck was this IVF stuff all about? The only thing I ever thought of when I heard IVF was "test tube baby." Boy, did we have alot to learn.

He Said...

Shortly after our engagement, amidst all our planning and calculations, I decided to surprise Debbie one day in an attempt to take some of the pressure off. I came home with airline tickets, hotel reservations and a week's itinerary for a trip to the big apple. I hadn't been there in over 10 years, and was yearning for a little big city fun and the possibility of a white Christmas. A week with Deb anywhere would be great, but I figured with her zest for life New York in particular would be a blast. Well I calculated right. Deb was ecstatic about a week in the apple. What I did not calculate and therefore became my first major step-parent-to-be blunder, was that now I had put her kids in the first, never before position of spending Christmas without their mom. We both rationalized that they were certainly old enough to spend a different kind of Christmas with their dad. Besides we were still going to spend Christmas together, just several days earlier . . . that was all. But anyway we sliced it, I had screwed up and Shannon would hold her grudge a little longer because of my misjudgment.

One afternoon we were having a particularly wonderful day

walking the streets of Manhattan when I suddenly got a brainstorm of an idea. Hey why don't we get married here? Now! Down at the courthouse. The hell with all the pre-rehearsed stuff. Let's elope, send the world a telegram and just have a big party afterwards when we got back home. Well it took Deb 5 ½ seconds to say, "How many blocks to the courthouse?" We found the courthouse and we were quite prepared to do it. But as fate would have it there was a room full of people waiting to tie the knot and it looked like at least a five-hour wait. I was starving, craving Chinatown grub so we decided to take off. In retrospect Debbie must have felt just a little bit passed over. After all I picked Lo Mein over *I do!*

The wedding day was one big fast forward; I remember looking sharp, feeling great, laughing, and singing. I was kissing people I never even met and before I knew it I was at the Port of Miami taking off for a week's cruise. If you were to write the text for a honeymoon, you could certainly model it after ours because we played the role perfectly. What a continuous high!

Six months into *newlywedness,* life's day to day realities had crept their way back into our lives. Deb had lost her job, we were still paying off two mortgages, and I was in a job that was like caster oil, necessary but hard to swallow. That August we learned that a reverse tubal ligation was not an option, and that in *vitro fertilization* was not a covered procedure in my medical plan. I was still not clear on what IVF really was, and with so many other things to worry about, I just placed it on the mental back burner.

By February Deb had landed a new job at a big medical company, we had sold her house in Coral Springs, Buddy decided to take roots up in Lakeland with his dad, and we had moved into my townhouse. The one thing about Deb and I, when we decide to strike, we move quick, swift, and leave a subtle cloud of smoke as a reminder. I was learning to digest corporate caster oil, and with a level of relative stability in our lives at that particular moment, we decided that now was as good a time as any to explore the path of clinical baby production. Might as well get it done now I thought. We were on a roll and we certainly wanted to knock this off the *To Do List* so that we could move on to all the other things that still needed to be done. "Okay," I said, "lets make an appointment and find out what this IVF stuff is really all about."

47

Chapter Three
So . . . What is This IVF Stuff?

She Said...

We made our appointment to visit with Dr. David again and find out what was involved with this thing called *IVF*. We were ushered into that same, unobtrusive office and an assistant popped a tape into the VCR that was supposed to explain the whole procedure. It sure did. I was scared to death. All those shots. All those drugs. *Yuck! Ouch! Maybe we should reconsider this?*

At the time we were in the program, the success rate for getting pregnant via IVF was only 25%. Not the best odds. When Dr. David imparted that fact on Eli, he was ready to leave. Not me. Despite my fear and loathing of needles, I wanted to know more. He said that I was probably a good candidate for IVF since I was only 35 years old at the time, and had already had two children. In other words, I'd already "proved" that I could have kids and I was still young enough to have them. But, he also stressed, as did Dr. Wayne, that there were absolutely no guarantees. Eli and I had already learned that lesson a long time ago!

Dr. David answered our questions as precisely as he could, without reservations, with sincerity and honesty. Eli still would have preferred guarantees but he was coming around.

An *in vitro fertilization* cycle takes approximately six weeks from beginning to end. Without a doubt it is the emotional roller coaster ride of your life. It can take you to the heights of rapture or plunge you to the depths of hell. It's definitely not for the emotionally weak. The IVF procedure is also one of the most expensive routes to child birth. A typical cycle costs between $8,000 and $10,000 including the hospital fees. Heavy tariff . . . but not that heavy when your goal is to hold a lightweight seven pounder!

Besides, we were among the "lucky" patients who had excellent insurance that would help defer the costs. My plan allowed for three IVF attempts and would cover 80% of the charges. If you didn't

49

achieve pregnancy after three tries . . . you were out of the game, or you'd better be prepared to further open your own wallet. We were grateful for the way my employment status had changed and that I was now working for a progressive company that covered this type of "let's get pregnant" option.

We listened with our mouths hung open and agreed to come back the following week for a "group" discussion to be held at the hospital. The group consisted of "IVF wanna-bes" and I instantly calculated that, according to the odds, only a few of us were going to be lucky enough to actually conceive a child this way. I ran into a couple that I had worked with at the computer company. They were contemplating IVF also. My thoughts were so selfish and I honestly felt guilty because if the odds were so low, then I wanted it to be *me who got pregnant*. The discussion was once again frank, open and honest. It focused on the mechanics of the entire IVF cycle, the drugs involved and their relative side effects, and the actual retrieval of the eggs and implantation of the embryos.

Eli and I spent alot of time at the library. We researched and read everything we could get our hands on. We read the book about the first *test tube* baby and giggled because there really wasn't any baby in a test tube! After months of discussion and evaluation, we finally decided to give it a shot. (The shots would be all mine of course, compliments of my husband!)

Contrary to my visualization of a "test tube baby," IVF can really be explained quite simply, without going into a clinical dissertation. It begins with stimulating your ovaries, using potent fertility drugs, to try to produce more than one egg per cycle. The eggs are then surgically "harvested" from the patient and fertilized with sperm in a Petrie dish, a small glass dish. Once the sperm fertilizes the egg, it becomes an embryo. After two to three days of allowing the embryo to grow and multiply into several cells, it is implanted into the uterus and hopefully becomes a baby. Simple, right? Yes and No.

The doctors go through a thorough dissection of your history and then perform any additional testing (laparoscopy, endometrial biopsies, etc.) that may be necessary to decide whether IVF is for you, or maybe some other option would suit you better. Once Eli and I were dissected to the point of distraction and our case was reviewed, we were informed that we could proceed with IVF if we chose to do so. Eli had to undergo quite a few tests too, which gave the doctors information they needed to know about how his sperm would react to my eggs. Could you imagine if they were "allergic" to each other?

Prior to entering our first IVF cycle, we were handed a rather

51

large pile of papers to sign. Consent forms. Consent to enter the program. Consent to perform the procedure. Consent to inject myself with Lupron. Consent to inject myself with fertility drugs. Consent forms for "after the operation" drugs. Consent form to freeze embryos . . . if you were lucky enough to have some left over to freeze. We joked that perhaps we should have brought a stamp with us and just stamped our name on all the forms. Signing the forms was the easy part especially since they let us take them all home and read and sign at our leisure. That was always one of the things I loved about this medical office, they never pressured you to do anything; every-thing was always at your own pace. You felt respected and somehow secure. And, no matter how many questions I had, or how dumb I thought they were, the doctors and nurses were always available to answer another stupid question and to put my fears at ease. Although the front office staff changed a few times, I became familiar with the primary IVF nurses: Debbie and Nancy who assisted Dr. David, and Justine who was Dr. Wayne's right hand. You quickly learn to trust those people who are sticking needles in you at regular intervals. They all had a professional, yet warm demeanor, but Debbie and Justine be-came my favorites. They held my hand and patted my shoulder more than once!

On one visit to the office, Debbie showed Eli how to give me a shot in my upper arm and in the muscle of my hip or thigh. I preferred my hip so I didn't have to see it go in my thigh. She used an orange to show how easy it was to accomplish and we also viewed a videotape. I took notes. Eli laughed . . . a little too sadistic for my taste!

The first step in an IVF cycle is to know when you ovulate. Debbie explained how critical this step was for proper timing of harvesting the eggs. I listened closely and committed to memory everything she told me but I was glad for the "Ovulation Timing" instructions and the calendar chart she gave me, preparing me for my first try. They also had a videotape available for me to review but I opted for the instructions. It was simple enough.

Using the calendar (that I taped up on the bathroom mirror where Eli usually shaved) and the Ovukit I could quickly predict when my ovulation day was. No brain scientists stuff here.

Once the doctors knew an ovulation date, they could calculate when to start the fertility drugs. The first step would be a shot of Lupron every day in my upper arm. That was an easy one . . . it was a tiny enough needle that I figured I wouldn't feel a thing. Lupron, in IVF cases, is used to prevent premature ovulation and it helped to produce uniform growth of my follicles. Follicles are the "water sacks" in which an egg grows. Lupron and various other fertility drugs are used to stimulate your ovaries and produce more follicles, hopefully with eggs in them. Most women produce one egg per month. We wanted a dozen.

Statistics say that a fairly high number of women (20% -50%) undergoing ovarian stimulation with fertility drugs alone, respond in an unsatisfactory manner. An LH surge and ovulation may occur. If this happened, then that particular IVF cycle would end and you would have to wait until the following cycle to begin again. Studies have shown that using Lupron in conjunction with the fertility drugs tends to avoid premature ovulation. Also, the number of eggs retrieved, fertilization rates, and implantation rates may be improved with the use of Lupron.

Okay, all right. So, I would take the Lupron.

Along with a shot of Lupron every morning, there would be a shot of Pergonal in the morning and a shot of Metrodin in the evening. Many factors are taken into consideration when the dosing for these drugs is determined. These fertility drugs are used to stimulate maturity of multiple eggs and to control their release at a predictable time. Harvesting, or collecting, the egg(s) is scheduled just before it's predicted to release.

I was told that once the drugs began, I would be in and out of the doctor's office routinely until the day of retrieval. Oh great… more time missed from work! I was already devising excuses as to why I would be late on a regular basis! Blood and urine tests would be taken regularly to monitor the growth of the follicles containing the eggs.

I found myself wondering what it would feel like to be a human pincushion. Would my arms be able to handle the constant stabbing of needles? Would I be so sore at the end of a cycle that they'd never be able to find a vein again? Would I ever be able to sit again? But, most importantly, would I be able to maintain my composure or would I be weak and break out in a cold sweat every time I had to have the blood test? I hate needles…would I survive this? Ultrasound exams provide a "picture" of the ovaries and provide a means for measuring the growing follicles. This part sounded like fun since I would be able see those little follicles growing, hoping there were eggs in them. But, there is a down side to this step. IF there aren't two or more mature follicles developing in response to the fertility drugs, you could be canceled from the cycle at this stage!

Once the doctors determine that the follicles are mature for harvesting, a date and time are scheduled for the hospital. Things move fairly quickly during this phase. Debbie or Justine would draw more blood, called the "media blood." Eventually, the serum obtained from this blood is used to supplement the culture medium. The nurses would also instruct me as to what time I would take an injection of HCG. HCG is used to stimulate the ovaries to release all their eggs.

When you arrive at the hospital, 34 hours after HCG, you are "prepped" and an IV is started. More needles. Under IV sedation, using either the laparoscopy or ultrasound guided retrieval method, the eggs are aspirated from the follicles through a long, thin needle. They're "sucked out" of the sack!

After confirmation that eggs have been retrieved from the follicles, a sperm sample is obtained from the husband. The sperm is "treated" in the laboratory to prepare it for fertilization. The eggs and the sperm are placed together in a special culture solution to allow fertilization to occur. After the eggs are fertilized, they are transferred into a culture dish with a solution necessary for growth.

Approximately two to three days later, you return to the hospital for the embryo transfer. It's usually a simple procedure of placing the embryo(s) into the uterus by means of a small tube inserted through the cervix. You can relax for a little while and then go home. Or, if you prefer, you can stay overnight in the hospital. Depending on the tilt and position of your uterus, you are instructed to either lie flat on your back or your stomach for 24 hours. No getting up. No moving around. No bathroom. You are immediately injected with a hefty dose of Progesterone to help support the lining of the uterus after egg retrieval. In an early study on in vitro fertilization, pregnancy rates improved once progesterone was utilized.

A blood test is taken ten days after the transfer to determine if you are pregnant. Ten days sounded like it was forever!

The above is the criteria that was followed by our doctors at that time. Other IVF programs may vary slightly, but this was the basic procedure we followed at the time we were in the program. It sounds like anyone who tries IVF should get pregnant . . . right? Well, despite reasonable precautions, any of the following can occur which would prevent the establishment of pregnancy:

* Ovulation timing may have been misjudged, or unpredicable, or ovulation may have already occurred, or may not occur in the monitored cycle, therefore preventing any attempt at obtaining an egg.
* Obtaining an egg can be unsuccessful.
* The egg(s) may not be normal, in which case they would not be transferred.

57

* The results of the blood and urine tests may show that the ovaries have had too little or too much stimulation and therefore you may be canceled from the cycle.

* The ultrasound may show no or only one developing follicle.

* The husband may be unable to supply a sperm specimen.

* Fertilization may not occur.

* Cleavage or cell division of the fertilized egg(s) may not occur.

* The embryo(s) may not develop normally.

* Implantation of the embryo(s) into the wall of the uterus may not occur.

* A laboratory accident may result in loss or damage to the fertilized egg(s) or embryo(s).

* Other unforeseen circumstances may prevent establishment of pregnancy.

The doctors also warn that even if pregnancy is successfully established, there is still the possibility of a miscarriage, ectopic pregnancy, stillbirth and/or congenital abnormalities. The risk of the development of an abnormal fetus was, at this time, unknown. From animal and human experience and from observations of the abortion of abnormal fetuses in the human, it is not now believed, that this procedure has any greater risk of abnormal fetal development than occurs in nature.

So, with all the risks and pitfalls that can happen along the road, is it worth it?

Absolutely!!

Chapter Four

The Male Ego Factor

He Said...

I am convinced that every man has an inner sexuality barometer buried deep within the bowels of testosterone, a sort of macho man report card that he keeps score on his conquests, his drive, his performance, so on and so forth. Some men insist on sharing their score with the world while others prefer to keep the results private. And then there are those who love to skew the numbers and portray themselves as god's gift. Regardless of which category we fall into, I truly believe that we all consider it an integral part of our manhood.

I prefer to side with those that chose to keep the results out of the tabloids. The truth is that I couldn't remember the names or the number of conquests I had achieved over the years if my life depended on it . . . a flaw that I was unmistakably proud of. Sex, in its raw sense was an act of pure pleasure, and on the thermometer of drive and desire, I was constantly running a 101° fever.

As you get older and more mature, pleasing your partner becomes equally as important, a sort of technical proficiency test you put yourself through, again in the ongoing quest to rate yourself. Well, in this category I suspected that I had gotten my initial certification and as far as I could read, I was getting my license renewed on a timely basis. Sure, there were the alcohol ridden nights that resulted in multiple apologies, or the occasional chemistry dysfunction with your mate, but all things being equal there were no problems in that department either. (Or so we all want to believe!)

So in typical left brain rationale, one plus one must certainly lead to two. In the new reproductive arena Deb and I were embarking in, the steps would be easy. I would sit back and hear the guidelines for IVF candidacy, but I wasn't really listening. After all, with all the ammunition I had already decided I was carrying, I couldn't imagine any situation under which the *male factor* would ever be a factor.

I distinctly remember the first time Dr. David's line of

questioning started to bother me. He had asked me if I had ever fathered a child before, to which I replied, "No." He stated that because I had not, it was necessary to test my sperm for suitability. *Suitability,* I said to myself, what's this guy talking about? I had not fathered a child in my life because I learned early in my adolescence that it was *not cool to knock up a broad!* And, given my previously poor marital situation, I had purposely insisted that my first wife stay on birth control pills. I was so taken by this line of insinuating questions that when he said I needed to make an appointment to give a sample, I wasted no time and volunteered to give a sample then and there, right on the spot! He said that such urgency was not warranted but I simply insisted. After all, my sperm had to be not only suitable but also superior as I remembered that 101° fever that I was harboring for so long. So after some discussion he agreed, and before I knew it I was in a cold examination room with a sterilized plastic cup in one hand, and . . . well . . . you know . . . something else in the other!

I remember walking out of the doctor's office that afternoon feeling like I had just recorded another notch in my belt. I was boasting to Deb what a piece of cake it was, and secretly thinking (for no explainable reason), what if all is not well in spermville? An hour later the whole thing was out of mind and life went on.

I had worked for my boss, Wayne, for the last seven years and was very comfortable with our relationship. Wayne is a very intense human being, totally devoted to the company and a true family man. Some managers feared him while the vast majority, at a minimum, were uncomfortable around him because of his drive and high level of expectation. I must have been in the clouds somewhere because I missed what everyone saw, and as a result not only was I not intimidated by him, but I actually enjoyed our professional relationship. I can't remember when, but at some point we also became friends, special friends, the kind that share private aspects of their lives with each other. Wayne had been my best man at our wedding and was very in tune with the components of my newly found life with Debbie. Consequently, I kept him up to date on my latest project: baby making.

Wayne and I had driven to Tampa together to attend a meeting and decided to check into a motel for the evening rather than make the five-hour trip back that same night. Before heading out for dinner I called Deb to let her know we were staying the night and to see what was new back home. We had conversed for about 15 minutes and I was trying to wrap up the conversation knowing that Wayne was waiting for me in the lobby. As I was trying to say good-bye, Deb after some hesitation, blurted, "The doctor's office called; the test results came back today."

"Oh yeah," I replied nonchalantly. "What did they have to say?"

She proceeded to give me a five-minute speech on technical terms that I was not comprehending. I finally interrupted her and said, "So what's the bottom line honey? Wayne's waiting for me downstairs."

I heard her draw in a deep breath before she said, "Well there seems to be a problem." To which I quickly replied, "Don't worry honey, whatever it is we can overcome it. They can give you fertility drugs, or . . . "

"THE PROBLEM IS NOT WITH ME!" she shot back.

"What do you mean the problem is not with you?" I asked with a defensive tone, getting ready to ask the follow up question but actually being afraid to do so.

"Who is the problem with?" As if I didn't know what the other choices were.

"Honey, they said something about this and something about that, and they said you needed to go in and get re-tested."

After repeated questioning Deb finally elaborated and shared with me that all aspects of the test seemed normal except that the sperm count was low. LOW, I screamed inside to myself, impossible! All those report cards, the constant 101° fever, the conquests! All of it.

It just couldn't be. There must be some mistake.

During dinner that evening, Wayne could have fired me, sold me the Brooklyn Bridge, or hit me in the face with his key lime pie, and I would not have realized it for 72 hours. All I could think about was: *where were all the missing sperm?* Were they playing hide and seek with the lab technicians? Did I misplace them somewhere? Heavens, maybe years of promiscuity had finally caught up with me, maybe I just ran out. Whatever the mystery, I couldn't wait to get back home to ask the trillion questions that were going through my mind. There had to be a reasonable explanation.

Later that week I was back in Dr. David's office trying to sort out all of the medical jargon and before I left I made another deposit for the good doctor so that he could have it tested again. In the meantime I was instructed to stay light on alcohol and cigarettes, and to try to avoid tight briefs. Somehow, through this entire inquisition, I managed to keep my sense of humor. I'll sit on a block of ice if I have to, I chuckled to myself. Yet, I knew I was fighting back pent up anger.

The following week I received a personal telephone call from Dr. David.

"The tests came back the same, the sperm count is still low," he said as if he were reading it from some rehearsed script.

"I want you to see a urologist as soon as you can," he told me.

"A urologist," I pleaded, "what on earth for?"

"Well one possible reason for the low count may be a varicose vein," he replied.

A *varicose vein,* I said to myself. I thought women in their 60's got those in their legs. By the time I hung up, I was feeling sick to my stomach and my face was quite pale. All sorts of thoughts raced through my mind. Where was the vein? Maybe I had a bigger problem; maybe it was testicular cancer. How did this happen? Was it something I did? Was it hereditary? By the end of the day I had lost all focus on IVF and I was convinced that I was fighting for my life.

The following Thursday I was in the urologist's office telling my tale to the doctor. I had been a patient of his in the past for a urinary tract infection once, and a prostate flare up twice so he had some history on me. After some conversation about the possible reasons for the low sperm count, he did a complete examination of my reproductive tools, reciting the results of his findings into a small tape recorder. He concluded the examination with a full prostate massage that yielded prostatic fluid, which he then would test to see if it had white cells (which would indicate a persistent and recurrent prostatitis).

During the follow-up consultation he reassured me that

everything that he visually inspected looked normal. He detected no signs of varicose veins, the sperm test was within normal parameters and as far as he was concerned, I was perfectly healthy. For the first time he offered a possible explanation to my dilemma: maybe I was just under alot of stress.

I was back in Dr. David's office the following week, feeling like a ping pong ball. I brought my entire test results and copies of the urologist's notes with me for his review. Dr. David looked somewhat perplexed as we discussed my situation. On one hand the IVF process had certain eligibility criteria from both the male and female perspective which he did not want to compromise, and on the other hand no definitive reason had been pinpointed for my situation.

I guess stress is that silent player that always takes the rap for things that are otherwise unexplainable in medical science, sort of a designated fall guy if you will. I was certainly inclined to believe that stress was a very possible culprit, after all I had plenty of it coming from all angles in my life. But I should have known that we were not going to write it off to stress and move on.

No sir. Dr. David had more tricks up his sleeve. He had another test he wanted to administer to test the performance of the limited number of sperm I was producing. This test was called the *Hampster*

Penetration Test. Put simply, they would unite my sperm with a hamster's egg to see if the sperm could penetrate the egg and begin the process of fertilization, just like the human process. You can imagine how excited I got at the prospect of having the opportunity to impregnate a hamster.

I was really beginning to resent this whole process. The preliminary test stage had turned into a circus of personal humiliation. Bad enough I was spending all this time in and out of doctor's offices, being poked, prodded, massaged, rated, giving samples, having Human Resources' personnel read my medical claims, and now on top of everything else, having to get this hamster pregnant. What if I couldn't do it? By now my manhood had taken a few hard hits, but the thought of not matching up to a male hamster, failing to rate at least equally to this member of the rodent family really had me down. Oh no . . . more stress, which equals less sperm, I better snap out of it!

That weekend Deb and I spent our time at the library reading everything we could get our hands on relating to infertility and the male involvement. The more I read the better I felt, as I was at least getting a more detailed picture of the pieces of the puzzle. Doctors typically do not have the patience to hold your hand and explain all the intricacies of a particular problem, or a possible problem, many times leaving you with a very empty feeling inside.

The material we found put things into perspective, and by the time we left I was convinced that I had to chill out, and make sure I had a damn good looking hamster!

I was in a pretty relaxed mood on the morning I went to provide yet another sample for the hamster penetration test. I remember thinking about all of the amusing sides of this encounter. What if the hamster didn't turn me on? Worse yet, what if it did, what would that signal? Suppose the procedure worked and the hamster got pregnant? Was I setting myself up for a paternity suit?

"Your honor I admit that this hamster is my responsibility, and I promise to meet all of my financial obligations, but please understand why I am relinquishing all my visitation rights." What if I gave the rascal up for adoption and 20 years later, the young adolescent hamster chose to find out who his real father was? As I played out all these scenarios in my mind, a lab technician approached me with a cup in hand and promptly announced, "Mr. Franco, it's your turn."

Two weeks later we were back in Dr. David's office to hear the results of the test.

"Well there was some penetration of the egg," he grimly told us. You could hear a pin drop afterwards. Deb and I looked at each other, not knowing whether we were supposed to be disappointed or elated about the results.

"Give it to me straight Doc, what's the bottom line?" I said.

By this time I had exhausted all my patience and was fed up with the whole charade. Dr. David looked at Deb, and as he scribbled some notes in our file, he said with a certain sense of proclamation, "The next IVF cycle starts in March if you guys want to get started."

"March sounds fine to us," we sang in absolutely perfect unison.

As we left the office, we were rambling about how we had finally gotten through this tough period. Driving back home, replaying the entire process from beginning to end, I couldn't help thinking in particular about the last phase of the process with the hamster penetration test.

Somewhere out there was a hamster, I thought, that I was capable of impregnating. Mentally I gave myself three high five's and like excess gas after a heavy meal I let loose on a YEAH! Deb looked at me, smiled and never asked me what that was all about. Somehow I suspected that she knew I was feeling just like old times. You know, maybe just a little feverish!

Chapter Five
The First Try

She Said...

All of the mandatory tests were done but before we could actually begin our first IVF cycle, we had to go through a "trial" transfer so the doctors would know the position of my uterus and be prepared for the real transfer of embryos when it was show time. We completed this quite easily and were "enrolled" in the March, 1990 IVF cycle.

I picked up all the drugs I would be taking for the next six weeks from the doctor's office. I walked out with a shopping bag full of various sizes of needles (ouch) to inject the drugs. I also had a bottle of Lupron, several six packs of powdered Pergonal, small vials of diluent, which is used to mix the Pergonal, a vial of HCG and a vial of Progesterone. I was ready!

Debbie told me which cycle day I was to start the Lupron and then when to start the Pergonal.

Eli gave me my first Lupron shot in the morning of the appointed day and we were off. He would also inject me with a shot of Pergonal every morning and night. He only drew blood a couple of times and after the first few days, he was a pro at injecting with minimal pain, and I had perfected the line: "It didn't hurt a bit!"

We were both so excited about the possibility of the end result. And scared too. So many drugs, so many possible side effects. But, I turned out to be the perfect patient. I had very few side effects and seemed to breeze through the whole procedure.

I didn't tell any of my co-workers that we were trying to have a baby because I didn't want to upset my still rather new job situation. Since I was considered the new kid on the block, and still trying to "prove" myself, I didn't want to upset any applecart, prematurely. But, we did tell our friends about this IVF stuff and some were skeptical. We believed that part of their skepticism came from their lack of knowledge, so we forgave them. Others were thrilled for us and would ask regularly about our progress. Some of their questions would make us shake our heads in wonderment. Although we thought it was as

72

simple as ABC's, in retrospect, I guess it's not an easy procedure to understand unless you are actually going through it.

So many people have misguided information about the "test tube baby" business. We took it upon ourselves to educate those who were interested and those who would listen. Most people mistakenly assume that they will always be able to get pregnant. They take it for granted that it will just happen . . . when they are ready to conceive. Although our particular situation was not due to infertility problems, the fact is that infertility rates are rising and this particular conception method is just one of many that offers hope to the childless couple.

And, hope we had. In fact, WE BELIEVED WE WOULD HAVE A BABY!

After the first two weeks on the drugs, I would show up at Dr. David's office for blood tests and an ultrasound to see how many follicles were developing. I made Eli go with me the first time I was scheduled to have an ultrasound because my nerves were a wreck. I was afraid I wouldn't have any follicles. Throughout the procedure, I prayed for five follicles. I wanted five because I thought, in some warped way, that it was a lucky number. There were already four people in our immediate family: Eli, Shannon, Buddy and me. The baby would make five!

It's funny how you lose all your inhibitions when you have higher goals in mind. At first, I was shy and reserved about having to do the "stir-up" routine on a daily basis but that quickly dissipated. I would get undressed, from the bottom down, in two seconds flat and be lying on the table, in position, waiting for the ultrasound to begin. I *wanted* to see my follicles! The heck with modesty.

We saw our first follicles together . . . all four of them and were thrilled that we had FOUR! That meant that we had four potential eggs and therefore, perhaps four embryos. Now, if we could just get through all of the steps, without getting canceled from the program, we would be home free. We were consumed with successfully reaching and overcoming each step without being "dropped" like a hot potato. We left the doctor's office, spirit's soaring and went to work. Eli called me later that day to see how I was feeling. I was doing great. He was afraid that the follicles were giving me cramps or something. The thoughts we had.

We met other couples that were also experiencing IVF for the first time. We would talk and compare follicle numbers and growth size while we waited our turn for either blood work or the ultrasound. I met a girl who came from Puerto Rico to try this procedure. She had 10 follicles! I couldn't believe it, but Dr. David said in his nonchalant way, "It happens." Oh. I went through the whole cycle with her . . . we even met in the hospital for retrieval on the same morning together. My husband and her husband bit nails together. She produced five eggs out of the ten follicles. Good odds, I thought. Her husband said they implanted all of them. We heard later that she didn't get pregnant and my heart ached for her.

My follicles were growing steadily, rapidly and were almost mature and ready for picking, or, "harvesting" as the doctors called it. When I would see the follicles on the ultrasound, they reminded me of plump black olives. First they were small, then medium and finally large ones.

One morning when I went to have my blood work and ultra-sound, Debbie told me it was time to take the "media blood." Media blood? What? She explained (again) that this was the blood they would use for the eggs and embryos during the retrieval and fertil-ization. I hated this part of the procedure as much as I hated an IV stuck in my hand. I had to lie on the bed while they took the required amount of "media" blood from me. I would sweat buckets and was always glad when it was over. It's not that it really hurt, it was just the anticipation of having it done. I couldn't look at it during or after-wards. I would hum to myself or talk gibberish to whoever was drawing the blood.

Okay . . . it's show time. With strict instructions not to eat or drink anything after midnight, Debbie told me to take my HCG precisely at 1:30 a.m. I set the alarm clock for 1:15 a.m. so Eli would be *awake* when he gave me the shot; I didn't want any goof ups at this stage of the game. I had nursed these follicles for six weeks and I wanted to make sure that we gave them the "push" at exactly the right time.

We went to the hospital the next morning for the retrieval process. I had emptied an egg carton to take with me and I planned on telling Dr. David to "fill it up," but Eli lost his sense of humor that morning and wouldn't let me bring it. We had been instructed to go to the third floor waiting room and a nurse would come to get us when they were ready. We watched *The Price is Right* on the small television set in the lounge area while we waited, and I must have gone to the ladies room ten times. Nerves. I was scared to death. Eli was chewing gum so I knew he was nervous too. We made up stupid egg stories to make each other laugh and to pass the time quickly. Thirty minutes passed before Justine came out, dressed in green scrubs, to retrieve us. No pun intended.

She took us down the hall to a cozy, intimate surgical room. I really mean cozy and intimate . . . the room was similar to the popular birthing rooms now found in hospitals everywhere. The lighting was dim and warm. The bed appeared to be a "normal" make and model. The dreaded stirrups weren't visible. . . yet! And there was a bathroom in the room . . . thank heavens because I had to go again.

We were given your standard hospital attire to change into: I got a white, open in the back, cloth dressing gown and Eli got blue scrubs that included a hat, face mask and shoe covers. I quickly changed and found myself shivering and shaking. Nerves. Justine tucked me into bed and found warm blankets to wrap around me. When Eli came out, dressed in his blues, I cracked up. His head was covered with this dorky hat, he had the facemask on already and he had the shoe covers on backwards. What a sight.

We sat in peace and quiet, holding hands for a few minutes until the action started. Before we knew it, people we had never seen appeared out of nowhere. They wheeled in all types of equipment that we couldn't fathom a use for. We just looked at each other with wide eyes that said it all. I was having seconds thoughts at this point. I wanted to go home and not do this after all. Even though we had been prepared for what would happen, we didn't know the reality of it all.

The next thing I knew, the anesthesiologist was introducing

himself and asking me how I felt. SCARED. He patted my hand and told me there was nothing to worry about. Sure. He had a great bedside manner and told us a few jokes in between asking me what I thought were pertinent questions. I had to go to the bathroom but I knew it was too late to ask. He asked me if I had anything to eat or drink after midnight.

"No, just toothpaste and a little water to rinse."

He asked me my weight and I lied to him. No way was I telling a room full of strangers what I weighed. It was one thing to have all those people in there while I was laying in a prone position with my legs in stirrups for the whole world to see, and another to have them all know my weight. Enough is enough. I figured it wouldn't matter in the long run anyway!

He prepped the top of my hand with a cleansing solution, found a vein and then gave me a shot that stung something awful. He told me the shot was only to numb my hand so he could insert the IV needle. Oh. Eli was sitting on my right side and I kept my head turned towards him while Dr. IV did his thing. I shivered and had to go to the bathroom.

We eavesdropped on the conversation taking place in this not so warm and cozy room after all, and realized that the cast and crew were part of the IVF lab at the hospital. They were the people who would be taking care of my embryos until they were implanted in me. I liked them better once I realized they were the caretakers of our future child.

Every now and then Justine would yell over to me: "How ya doing' Deb?"

"Great, just great." It dawned on me then that it was JUSTINE who was in the room . . . not Debbie. Since Justine was the other half of Dr. Wayne, did that mean that Dr. David wasn't going to be here? Geez . . . I had only met Dr. Wayne once. I was "officially" Dr. David's patient and saw him regularly. Where was Dr. David? Just before I could voice my concerns to Eli, in walked Dr. Wayne . . . smiling and ready to go. After a few minutes of chitchat, things progressed quickly. Okay, Okay, I'll take Dr. Wayne. What choice did I have?

The nice, comfortable, warm bed I had been laying in was efficiently turned into a surgical table with stirrups that magically appeared from the bottom of the bed and an extension of the bed was pulled out from me feet. Here we go.

I was given an oxygen mask that I immediately hated. I felt claustrophobic and begged to have it removed. They complied. I saw Dr. Wayne sit on a stool that was positioned at the foot of my bed. I could tell he was smiling because the apples of his cheeks pushed up his glasses when he said to me, "Not to worry, let's go to work."

He made me feel calm, safe and secure with such simple words. Okay . . . I'll take Dr. Wayne! The anesthesia, which was only Valium, hit me like a rock. I was out in a matter of seconds.

Eli watched on a monitor while Dr. Wayne expertly aspirated my four follicles. He was intrigued by the whole procedure and gained a new respect for this exacting science. The retrieval couldn't have taken more than 35 minutes. Done. I was slowly coming around and couldn't believe I had slept through the whole thing! It was over? That was it? Great, take this IV out now, please! Eli and I were thrilled with our accomplishment. Each precious follicle released its contents and we produced four eggs!! YEAH for us. Now for the next crucial step.

Eli was sent over to the doctor's office to spend some time in "the room" where he would produce the sperm to fertilize the four eggs. A nurse appeared to inject me with a shot of Progesterone, which is a tough drug to take. It's an oil-based serum and isn't easy to absorb into one's buttocks. Another ouch!

I fell asleep and woke up when Eli returned, apparently successful! I was awake enough and felt fine but they made us stay another hour to be sure all my vital signs were normal before releasing us.

The next step was to take Eli's sperm and put it together with the eggs for fertilization. And I was to continue taking Progesterone shots once a day. These shots proved to be a major pain in the butt. The stuff is so thick that you'd swear it would never absorb into your system. I wound up getting huge "balls," the size of a plum pit, underneath my skin at each injection site. I couldn't sit well because they hurt so badly and I walked sort of funny. A few of my co-workers thought I had hemorrhoids and that's why I had trouble sitting and walking. That theory worked well for me since I had been out of work for a few days, so I let them believe that and even encouraged it a bit. It was so far from the truth that it was actually funny to me too!!

We waited at home for one of the nurses to call us and tell us whether fertilization had occurred. It was an agonizing wait. What if they didn't fertilize? What if they fertilized but didn't multiply into several cells? What if ALL four of them fertilized? Did we want all of them implanted or should we freeze a couple? "What ifs" were all we did that day.

We both jumped for the phone. We fertilized. But, only two of the four. We had a 4-cell embryo and a 2-cell embryo. Okay . . . we'll take the two, that's fine, Okay. Another hurdle mastered. We hugged and kissed and acted like two kids who had just been told they could have a puppy.

We were scheduled to return to the hospital the following day for the implantation. Once I knew we were going back into the hospital for the transfer, I stopped drinking all fluids. I wouldn't be allowed to get up for 24 hours and there was no way that I was going to use a bedpan! We could hardly sleep that night. We just wanted to go to the hospital and get our embryos.

The transfer took all of ten minutes. Easy. Simple. No shots. No pain. Dr. Wayne transferred both embryos back into me and I said a small prayer and kept my fingers crossed that they became babies. Since we planned on having two kids, we hoped that this IVF attempt would result in twins. How lucky could we get?

Immediately following the transfer, I was wheeled into a bright, pleasant hospital room where I would spend the next 24 hours lying flat on my stomach. This was murder on my back but I figured I could tough it out. I wasn't going to complain. The end was in sight. Or rather, a new beginning!

Eli went out and got us some lunch, even though the hospital had plenty of food to offer. Ah . . . no thanks. I ate the sandwich but refused the soft drink. I was already *thinking* about going to the bathroom! This had to be a mind over matter thing and I planned on winning. I'd brought a novel with me but it was impossible to read in that position. The room was equipped with both a TV and VCR so we watched a few movies in between our daydreaming talks.

Shannon came up to the hospital that evening and although she wasn't thrilled about our baby making plans, she offered her support and stayed to watch movies and eat dinner with us. Our excitement returned and we were filled with anticipation and joy for what the future offered.

We left the hospital the next morning and tried to resume our normal lives. We went to work as usual, swam in the pool on weekends, went to the movies, and had dinner with friends. We had to mark off ten days before we could return to the doctor's office for a blood test to find out if we were pregnant. Around the eighth day I started to get a cold. My nose was stuffy and I just generally didn't feel good. My breasts were achy also but I didn't think anything of it. We were tempted to buy a home pregnancy kit but decided against it since it probably wouldn't be able to give accurate results that early in a pregnancy.

On the tenth day, nervous and excited, I went for the blood test and it was the first time I had willingly shared my veins in six weeks. I left the office and went to work with a promise from Nancy that they would call me in the afternoon with the results. I almost told her to wait and call me after work at home but I knew Eli would be waiting for my call so I didn't. Every time my phone rang that day I found myself pressing my ear closer to the receiver anticipating hearing one of those familiar voices. It was nerve-racking. I didn't want to talk to anyone else. I just wanted someone, *anyone* from Dr. David's office.

Eli called around 2:00 p.m. to ask if they had called me yet. "Yeah, they called hours ago and I'm deliberately not calling you so you'll go nuts waiting like I am!" I knew he was just as anxious as I was but they hadn't called so I didn't have anything to report. He reminded me, for the umpteenth time, that if he wasn't in his office to beep him. I know, Dear!

I was completely absorbed in a marketing project when the call came at 3:00 p.m. that afternoon.

"Debbie Franco," I answered in my at-work, professional voice.

"Debbie, this is Nancy from Dr. David's office."

"Hold on Nancy while I close my office door," I told her.

"Hi Nance . . . how are you?" I asked her. Like this was a nonchalant call from a friend!

"I'm doing great . . . how are YOU feeling?"

"Fiiiiine," I replied.

"Well, are you sitting down?" She asked. "Yes, I am." Come on . . . let's get this over with. My adrenaline was pumping. My heart was in my mouth, I could barely breathe and we were chitchatting!!

"I've got good news for you . . . you're pregnant." I could picture her smiling and heard her laughing.

"Oh my God . . . are you sure?" was my dumb comment. Of course they were sure. I started laughing and crying all at the same time and thanked her profusely. It was overwhelming joy. All the stress, the emotional upheaval, the worry . . . it was all worth it for that very moment and those two words: "You're pregnant." I hung up the phone and kept trying to wipe my tears away. I needed to get a grip before someone in the office saw me and before I made the phone call to my husband.

I picked up the phone and dialed his office. His secretary must have been put on alert for my call because he was on the phone before I could even ask for him!

"Hi hon . . . it's me.

"Hi . . . did they call?" he asked.

"Yes sweetie . . . they called. Looks like you're going to be a Daddy!"

"What? What did you say? Oh. Oh WOW!" My husband, who is never at a loss for words, was absolutely dumbfounded and ecstatic. I remember laughing and crying again and we were both babbling idiots as we said, "Goodbye, see ya tonight, love ya," and hung up the phone. After I regained my composure again, I called a few of my friends and told them the news. Everyone was thrilled. It worked. We were going to have a baby. WOW!!

Shannon, Eli and I went to an Italian restaurant that evening to celebrate with milk and pasta. We talked and laughed and ate and made plans for the future. We had to get out of that townhouse . . . there just wasn't room for us there, not now with the new baby coming.

By the next day, EVERYONE knew we were pregnant *except* my co-workers! They still thought I had hemorrhoid problems! We basked in the congratulations with thousand watt smiles pasted on our faces. My concentration level wasn't what it should have been at work and several times I caught myself lost in thought with a stupid grin on my face. Our plans for that Friday evening included dinner with Eli's parents so we could let the prospective grandparents fawn over us.

However, we had to cancel our dinner plans that evening because by the time I got home from work, I was bleeding. Eli called

Dr. David's office and the answering service picked up. He told them
it was an emergency and a nurse called us back. He explained the
situation and she informed him of the probable outcome. I was sitting on the couch praying and crying my heart out. Eli tried to console
me but I was in no mood. Just let me cry. Let me mourn because I
already knew that I was having a miscarriage. I would never hold this
little baby in my arms or smell that sweet baby smell. I'd never get to
cuddle her or rock her to sleep. Oh yes, I was sure it was a baby girl!
I wished we had never told any of our friends about this. I didn't want
the sympathy or the "you can try again," comments. I had horrible
cramps that reinforced the inevitable and I just wanted to get it over
with and move on. We each mourned in our own way that weekend. I
cried streams full and Eli nursed his pain by walking on the beach . . .
alone. We held each other on Sunday and promised that after we
recovered we would try again because we were both determined to
have a child. But, for now, we needed to rest, to heal and relax. We
agreed to get off the roller coaster ride for a little while at least.

    I went to the doctor's office on Monday so they could take
another blood test to confirm what we all knew. They were sad for me.
Justine hugged me; she didn't need to say anything. I left there thinking how hard it must be for all of them. They see women everyday

who are on the quest for a baby. Some are rewarded with that tiny infant and some aren't. It must be gratifying to them when they are successful in helping to bring a child into the world and hard for them also to see the pain etched into so many faces when the procedure fails to produce the coveted reward.

We moved on in typical Debbie and Eli fashion and threw ourselves into another project. This time we were determined to dump the townhouse and get the heck out of there. It was time for us to have "our" house. I wanted a "real house" with green grass everywhere in the front and back of our house. We needed closet space, we needed breathing space.

We didn't list the townhouse with a broker again. Instead, we decided that drastic measures were needed. We created flyers to advertise the townhouse and put them in the windows of local stores. Wherever there was an open bulletin board in Dade or Broward County, we posted our flyer. We offered a "finder's fee" to anyone who found us a buyer. We gave a sales pitch to any prospective buyer who would listen to us. In the end, it took creative financing on our part but we finally sold that townhouse to a newly married couple who didn't have a down payment, but were a good financial risk. It took us a year to sell it! Once we had the contract signed, we really started looking for a house.

He Said...

IVF is no different from cars or true loves. You always remember your first.

Now that I had gotten past the sperm thing with confidence fully restored, I was ready to do my part. I gave Deb her shots, followed all the rules and put up with alot of abuse the first several weeks. Some of the initial drugs that Deb was taking were having a wee bit effect on her. Apart from some of the babbling she was doing, mood swings were common. GREAT, I thought, I'm getting a little insight into what life might be like 25 years from now.

I tried to be as tolerant and supportive as possible since she was the one enduring all of the physical sacrifice. Things were moving along quite well. With each doctor's visit, came a new follicle report card . . . 6 mm, 9 mm, 12 mm, boy can those follicles grow. I remember one day walking on the beach while Deb was at the doctor's office, going through her early morning routine. The thought of not knowing the progress that my son or daughter had made until later in the day was unacceptable so we devised a system using my pager. Sure enough around noon that day, while walking on the boardwalk, the pager went off and there in plain view were the numbers: 14, 16, 19, and 18. With a huge smile and immediate check to see if anyone was watching me, I proceeded to have my own little celebration. "A Miller Lite, my good man and start me a tab."

When *D-Day* arrived, I was ready. Not only to continue with the procedure, but I was more than ready to produce a sample. One of the stipulations during the cycle was no sex . . . two to three days before retrieval. So when the nurse presented me with my cup and escorted me to the room, I was fully prepared to do my baby-making duty.

The two-day wait that followed was probably a little harder for me than Deb because I single handedly proclaimed myself responsible for the outcome of fertilization. The day the doctor's office called and said that fertilization had occurred nicely, I was happy for us naturally and at that point felt fully vindicated of the charges bestowed upon me.

Your honor, on the one count of deficient sperm, we the jury find the defendant NOT GUILTY!

Yes sir, I was really rolling now. I felt like Superman; what a stud! Because you see, I, like only a select few, had proven that under the most clinical of circumstances I could produce offspring.

After the transfer of the two fertilized eggs, we went home

the next day where we had to wait ten days for an answer on the outcome. We seemed to be holding up well through the process until the last couple of days when the anxiety was starting to get really intense. Through our entire experience, I kept those people closest to me up to date on our cycle. Depending on whom I was talking to, I found myself dealing with varying degrees of explanation and clarification. My parents, who when it was all said and done would be supportive no matter what, were still not entirely clear on all of the mechanics of this process. I would patiently describe the step-by-step details to them. But something told me that it all had not sunk in yet. The truth is that most of the people we spoke to did not fully understand what IVF was all about either. Oh well, I thought, as long as they are praying for us, that's all that matters.

When Deb called to congratulate me that Wednesday after - noon, because I was going to be a daddy, I thought I could walk on water. Sharing the news with my inner circle was gratifying because I was about to become part of "the club." But, by Friday evening it was becoming apparent that my membership application was being rejected. Although the nurse told me over the phone to keep Deb off her feet for the weekend, and to have her go to the office first thing Monday morning, I sensed that things were not going to turn out right.

Sure enough by mid-week, the doctors had confirmed our suspicions. Deb had miscarried.

I thought the news about entering fatherhood had been a pretty well kept secret at work. But, as in most organizations, leaks are common and I remember receiving a Father's Day card as an expression of congratulations. How ironic that I received the card in the interoffice mail on the same day that the doctor's office had called to confirm the miscarriage.

Chapter Six
Round Two

He Said...

House hunting was occupying a significant portion of our time. We had just completed a domino real estate transaction where we sold, bought, resold, and financed a piece of property through our real estate corporation. Now we were positioned to buy our primary residence. We searched for nearly a year, and like so many things in our lives, our dream house came quite by accident.

We were looking for a particular open house in Pembroke Pines one Sunday afternoon but could not seem to find the correct address. After making a wrong turn, we stumbled upon a house that had just been placed on the market that weekend through a *Buy-Owner* agent. We entered the house, looked around a bit, looked at each other and could tell immediately that this was the house for us. Deb and I went outside and talked about the possibilities. There I was trying to decide how I was going to negotiate the price down, and my wife trying to figure out what color furniture we needed to buy in order to match the decor. We both do have a few qualities that are typical, though not very many. Three hours later we had agreed in principle on the terms of the purchase. I remember vividly, as I was writing the seller the good faith check as part of the initial down payment, the feeling of the fourth bedroom. The couple we were buying the house from were empty nesters, the kids being out on their own for some time. The fourth bedroom was decorated as a nursery complete with furniture. Being grandparents, they had set up the room for their granddaughter's visits. I was convinced that this was an omen, a message from higher up saying, "You're going to need this fourth bedroom someday. Hey, by the way here's a present, it's already decorated and ready for use." We knew this was the house for us!

Although we closed on the house in August, we weren't planning to move until the sellers finished building their new home. They estimated their home to be ready around the first of the year.

With renewed vigor and hope we enrolled in the fall IVF cycle. We felt if nothing else a bit more relaxed about beginning the process simply because we had already gone through it and pretty much knew what to expect. Both Deb and I were more settled in our respective jobs which made for less career stress at a time when stress was forbidden. Deb went one afternoon to pick up her Ovukit so that she could get a pulse on her ovulation timing. When she arrived at the office, she was nonchalantly informed that Aids testing was now a requirement before the cycle actually began. I felt like I had just had the Gatorade cooler dumped on me in sub-zero weather.

When Deb and I decided to get married, back in 1989, we found out, much to our surprise, that a blood test was no longer required when applying for a marriage license. So, that led to a very intimate conversation about our past one afternoon in our bedroom . . . over a bottle of wine.

Sort of an Eli before Deb, and Deb before Eli talk.

I remember when we discussed the subject of Aids Deb was not particularly concerned about it. In 1989 public ignorance still prevailed and Aids was a *gay man's* disease. The first signs of hetero-sexual transmission were beginning to gain notoriety right about then. Deb reassured me that she had not led a promiscuous life during

95

the years after her divorce and she confidently stated that there was nothing to worry about. I, on the other hand, potentially had plenty to worry about. The latest medical reports were showing that incubation periods could be as long as ten years for this new plague of the 90's. Increasingly heterosexual transmission was becoming more and more of a viable segment of the infected population. Well I could not, and would not want to try to, remember every reckless encounter that I had over the last ten years. Suffice to say that I had certainly increased my odds because of the number of different partners over the years. We had both decided back then that since a blood test was not necessary then we weren't going to open Pandora's box. The matter was closed.

Now, 18 months later, fate had it that for entirely different reasons we would have to reconcile the acts of our past. Content with not knowing just wasn't good enough. If there was a cat in the bag, it was going to have to come out. So 48 hours after the news hit, the anxiety still fresh in our minds, there we were having blood drawn at the doctor's office. The office said that the results would be back in *several* days. Around day three I was really starting to feel uneasy about the whole thing. Thoughts of payback entered my mind. Punishment for all the wrong I had done in my life. What a sentence. What an embarrassment. What would people think? My friends, my family.

I began to draw up a plan, because you see I am a man that always has a plan, always! If we tested positive our life would take a whole new direction. We would obviously not have children; we would focus on entirely different things. For one, we would quit our jobs and travel. We would turn our entire net worth into liquid cash and see the world. Second, we would not tell anyone what had happened or why such a radical change in lifestyle. But then came the real knife in the heart, hair-raising thought. What if only ONE of us tested positive and the other one was okay? How would we survive that? Could our marriage survive that? The thoughts were starting to take their toll on us. First a week had gone by, and then it was 10 days and still no answer. Surely the delay must have meant that they were retesting the blood work because there was a problem. I was sure we were doomed. Finally I asked Deb to call and find out. When she did, the answer was unbelievable. The blood work had just gone out to the lab that afternoon. It seems that the office waited until they had the blood work of all the couples in the cycle before they sent them out in batches to the lab. Boy was I mad! Steaming mad! Why didn't they tell us this at the beginning? Ten days of planning your death only to learn that the test had not even been done yet. They assured us the results would be back in 72 hours. The only problem was that there was a weekend involved so it may not be back until the later part of the following week.

We had certainly learned by now that stress was not good for you during the cycle. Time and time again the doctors and nurses repeated that we had to try to minimize stress. Well they sure weren't helping matters any with this Aids testing. I do not believe I have ever been as stressed about anything as I was about this. By Friday I couldn't function very well. We both felt that this would be the day we would hear from the doctors. I remember telling Deb that morning not to call me at work with the results. I did not want to risk the possibility of coming unglued in front of my employees, peers or boss. No way. Wait until I get home.

Around 4:00 p.m. I really started to feel nauseous. You see, knowing my wife like I do, I figured that if the news was good, there was no way she wasn't going to call me. And since she had not called, the news had to be bad. I could not believe this was happening. So I picked up the phone and called her.

"They haven't called yet," she said hurriedly. "Hang up, I don't want my line tied up if they call." "Bye."…"Bye," I replied. My heart was pounding so hard, I swear I thought I was going to have a massive heart attack. How ironic if the test came back negative and then I died from a massive heart attack.

Finally at 4:50 p.m. my phone rang. Before I could finish identifying myself the voice on the other line was screaming, "We're OKay, we're OKay. We're not going to die, we're not going to die!" My God, I could not believe it. Immediately I thanked the Lord, and made one of those pacts you make when you luck out. You know the *I'll never ever, ever* type of resolutions we all make. Well this called for a celebration. Deb and I celebrated with pizza and a good bottle of wine!

She Said...

After one long, grueling Saturday of traipsing through new housing developments that weren't turning us on for one reason or another, we stumbled into a community that we hadn't seen but had driven past hundreds of times. We were driving around the neighborhood and had a good feeling about it. It just "felt like a neighborhood." Beautiful tree-lined streets, houses that didn't all look alike, kids riding bikes. Yards. We turned down a street and saw a "For Sale By Owner, Open House" sign. Eli wanted to go in but I was too tired to look anymore. "Let's come back tomorrow," I said. But, there was no detouring Eli. We rang the bell and walked into our dream house.

We both knew it immediately. It was a gut instinct and we both felt it.

As we walked through the house, we were giving each other the knowing looks. We walked through a second time and I knew I wanted this house. I began my sales pitch as we surveyed the outside perimeters of the house. On the sidewalk in front of the house, I very emphatically told my husband, "This is THE HOUSE for us; go in there and make the deal!" He had no choice but to agree with me. There was no doubt that this house had "Franco" written all over it.

We signed the contract that evening and agreed to rent the house back to the owners until their new home was built . . . approximately three to four months. We could wait. Talk about excited. We could hardly stand it.

Driving past the house and touring our new neighborhood became a new routine for us. One Sunday afternoon we decided to drive my in-laws past the house to show them our next residence. We actually got bold enough to bang on the door and ask if we could take a quick peek to show mom and dad. These people were so warm and gracious. They not only let us come in and show off our new home, they invited us for coffee and said we could come back any time to measure rooms or do whatever we needed to do.

We decided the time was right to begin our baby pursuit again.

I went to pick up my supplies and I found out that we had to have an AIDS test before we would be able to enroll in the next cycle. No big deal, or so I thought.

Eli was bongos about the test. Apparently he had really been a Don Juan in his past life and was scared to death about knowing the results of his wandering . . .um, eyes! Nevertheless, he consented to the test and then drove me absolutely nuts while we waited for the results. He was convinced he was going to die. I wasn't particularly worried about it and I tried to keep him calm, but he was a nervous wreck.

When we finally did get the results, he wanted to celebrate and of course, I shared his enthusiasm. We drank a bottle of wine and ate too much pizza that night, but we were deliriously happy!

Time was passing quickly but before we started our next IVF cycle, we wanted to relax and enjoy life. Shannon would be spending Thanksgiving with her dad and Eli and I had been invited to spend the holiday in Iowa, with long time friends, Joan and Armando. Joan's parents still lived in her hometown, Tabor, Iowa and welcomed us with open arms. We decided to fly to Boston first and tour some of the New England states and then fly to Iowa to meet up with our friends.

As usual, we had a blast in New England and were thrilled with having Thanksgiving in a small town that still left their doors unlocked at night. Eli was actually considering moving to this town and one day all of us were in the local tavern, shooting pool and drinking a few beers when Eli asked the bartender what kind of employment possibilities there were in Tabor. "Well," she said with a long drawl, "They're opening up a new Wal-Mart and they're lookin' to hire over there." As we all collapsed in laughter, I could see by the look on Eli's face that he was indeed contemplating it and wondering how to sell me on the idea! There was no sale to be made!

We were feeling quite relaxed and satisfied with life when we returned from that trip and decided it might be time for round two of our baby making adventure. We contacted Dr. David and made the arrangements to pick up our IVF drugs and set about on the roller coaster ride once again.

Eli gave me the drugs as normal, I had my routine checks at the doctor's office and basically everything was going along as planned. We retrieved two eggs, which both fertilized without any problems and I had them implanted into my womb without incident. Without anything.

After a few days, Eli started to ask me if I had any "symptoms." Nope. Nothing. He was dog faced. I was dejected. I went for my blood test on the tenth day, as scheduled, but I knew I wasn't pregnant. In retrospect, we should have waited awhile longer. We were still defeated from round one and round two had no excitement or optimism. We were just going through the motions. We expected defeat.

We moved on...looking forward to something that we could control: moving into our new house.

Chapter Seven
Three Strikes & You're Out?

She Said...

We finally closed on the house and took our keys to go look at our new, empty home. We sat quietly on the floor of the family room and looked at each other with stupid grins on our faces. We did it. Determination and perseverance once again paid off for us.

We moved into our home and started settling down again . . . this time for a longer period of time! The house seemed so big to us at the time. We had all that furniture that we practically gave away and now we had to go shopping for all new furniture to fill this house. I had tons of energy for that job!! In fact, I threw myself into furniture shopping on a regular, weekend basis. It helped to dull the pain of two attempted IVF cycles with no positive results.

I measured rooms and took samples of fabric back and forth to furniture stores. We were extremely lucky that the former owners had very good taste and our window treatments were all in fine shape and didn't need to be replaced. The Berber carpeting was also practically brand new so we decided to keep it for awhile. I took stock of each room and mentally knew what I wanted; it was just a matter of finding everything. The first thing we did was buy a new bedroom suite and it was delivered just before we formally moved in. We decided to turn one bedroom into Eli's office (I don't know how I let him convince me that it was HIS OFFICE!), so we just needed office furniture in there. Easy enough. Shannon took the front bedroom and I let her have free reign in decorating. We went shopping and she picked out new verticals and valances to match along with lamps, wall hangings, pillows and a beautiful comforter. She was finally "coming around" and starting to accept my marriage and not resent Eli's intrusion. I actually heard her laughing with him at times and talking candidly about her work or school activities. He helped her put up the new blinds and arrange her room the way she liked it. I finally felt at peace with her and thanked my husband more than once for giving her the space she needed to observe him and accept him for the good person he really is!

105

The last bedroom was already decorated for a baby girl. The wallpaper was a delicate print of tiny rosebuds and violets and the room would be perfect for the little baby I longed to put in there.

I finally decided on the formal areas and picked neo-modern black and white furniture and used mauve and seafoam greens for color. We chose a casual set for the family room since we knew that we'd be hanging out in there more often than not. It didn't take too long to furnish the house and make it into our home. I was itching for a new project again.

It was an early summer morning when I went to the train station to pick up my son. He was spending the summer with me and then heading back to his dad's for the school year. It was so good to see him. He had just turned 16 and was already taller than his father. And boy could he eat. We settled him in the "spare" bedroom, gave him a few curfew rules and then let him loose to go surfing with his friends. He was only home for two days when his father sent me a letter telling me that he didn't want Buddy to come back to live with him. He was having all of Buddy's possessions delivered to me that following weekend. Buddy had no idea what was happening and was under the impression that he would be returning to his dad's at the end of summer. I was furious at his father for just "dumping" him like that and not even bothering to tell him ahead of time. He left that little detail up to Eli and me. Buddy was also doing so well in the schools in Lakeland and I didn't want to rock that boat! I was scared to death to put him in the high school he would have to attend here. He would have to be bussed to the school and I knew Bud wouldn't like that at all. We couldn't afford a private school for him either. We were going to have to take our chances with the local high school.

Eli and I had a long discussion about how to break the news to my son and in the end, only the truth would work. We sat him down one evening and explained the situation to him. He was totally upset, to put it mildly. It hurt. I knew he was feeling rejected and hurt and angry all at the same time. He just kept asking me: "WHY?" I told him he would have to ask his dad that question. He refused to talk to his father. He was a walking time bomb . . . restless and ready to ex-plode at any minute. It was difficult to talk to him about anything after that.

We enrolled him in school, but he rarely went. His grades fell immediately. His principal called me so often that he had me on speed dial. I talked, yelled, cajoled and threatened my kid constantly. It was a losing battle. I finally took him to a psychologist so he could talk to an impartial, third party. It seemed to help him come to grips with his anger and frustration. He was angry with everyone by then!

I wanted to minimize his pain over the rejection I knew he must have been feeling and I told him the "spare" bedroom was now his. Of course he hated the beautiful tiny rosebud wallpaper. I didn't expect him to really like it anyway. Once again we were out shopping for furnishings for a bedroom. I let him decorate the room the way he wanted. Even though Eli and I hated what he did to it, we didn't say a word or deny him his right to fix up his room anyway he chose. He painted all the walls a dark chocolate brown and we used an even more morbid wallpaper border. His bedding was also in the dark family and all I could figure out was that these choices were indicative of the way my son was feeling.

We fell into somewhat of a routine and continued with our daily lives! But, the tension and stress were there.

Our first Christmas in the new house was wonderful, despite some of the problems we were having. We bought a new tree and the kids did the decorating. We hung mistletoe and had friends over for holiday parties. Everyone seemed to be settling down into our new life and our new surroundings so we started to talk about having a baby again. This would be our third try and the last one that would be covered under insurance. It had to work this time. We decided to wait until I had completed some important projects at work and a few of the critical trade shows were over.

Before we knew it, it was already May and we hadn't talked about number three at all.

It was time to go for it so I scheduled an appointment with Dr. David and went to talk about which protocol we would use this time. Because of two previous tries, they had been able to gather more information about me that could be useful in determining different dosages of drugs, and different protocols to use.

Although I was excited about trying again, something was missing. I could feel it. Maybe it was just all the stress we had been through in the past few months, or maybe it was the fact that we were losing our hope. We just weren't as UP as we had been. But then again, you can only take so much disappointment before you start putting your defenses up in an effort to protect yourself from the emotional roller coaster.

We started IVF cycle number three in May of 1991. We decided not to tell anyone, except our immediate family, about this attempt since we didn't want any prying questions or sympathy statements if we failed again. Maybe that was what was bothering us. We had failed twice. Neither of us are quitters. Neither of us are failures.

109

Everything we've ever attempted to do in life we've succeeded at. Damn it. *Why* couldn't we succeed at this? Didn't we want it bad enough? Reflecting back on the thoughts I was having during this cycle and the way I was behaving, it probably wasn't a good time to go through number three. There were so many other things on my mind . . . why was I doing this? Yet, I persevered. It seemed almost senseless. We had started believing that we'd lost. We were defeated already.

A few days before we were to begin the shots, Eli came home and told me he had to leave for Boston on a business trip. Oh, great. Now what? Who was going to give me the shots?

We considered asking his mom but since I had to have injections every morning, it was really too far out of my way to go to her house early in the morning . . . before work! We thought about Shannon, but no way could she handle it. She faints at the sight of a needle! I called a close friend and begged her to do it for me. She was squeamish but in the end agreed when she heard the desperation and panic in my voice.

So, for the first week I would drive to Judy's house early in the morning, get shot up and then make the trek to work. I'd leave the house at 6:15 a.m., get to Judy's at 6:45 a.m., and be back on the road at 7:00 a.m. with just enough time to arrive at work by 8:00 a.m. When I left work, I would make the journey back to Judy's house so she could give me my evening dose and I'd usually get home by 7:15 p.m...exhausted. It was a grueling week. I kept asking myself whether it was worth all the trouble. It wasn't good mind space at all!

I started the shots without much enthusiasm. I knew the routine. The shots were nothing to me now. "Yeah . . . yeah . . . just stick it in Judy, it's no big deal!" I would go to the doctor's office for my blood tests and ultrasounds and I wouldn't talk to the other patients like I had done previously. I just didn't feel like comparing notes. I didn't want to hear about how many follicles they had or how many attempts they had made. I didn't care anymore. Maybe, subconsciously, I was trying to not care so that I could fool my body into getting pregnant. *Hey . . . I don't care if you get pregnant or not. You don't want to . . . that's just FINE with me!* Maybe if I didn't care so much, it would happen. When I went in for my first ultrasound, there were no follicles to be found. Zilch. Zippo. None. Oh great . . . we're off to a wonderful start aren't we? However, as I continued to take the drugs, we started to see the formation of the follicles. I wound up with four follicles this time. I was thrilled. Four was good. That meant four chances for eggs and four chances for a baby.

111

Once again I met Dr. Wayne in the operating room. He was in fine spirits that day and wished Eli and me good luck. Yup…we wished ourselves good luck. I went night-night on a combination of Demerol and Valium. When I woke up, I found out that only two of the follicles produced eggs. Well, I'd been there before so I didn't think two was too awfully bad. We went home that afternoon and knew that we had to wait at least 24 hours before we'd receive a call telling us whether we fertilized or not.

The next day we got the call that both eggs had fertilized. YES! We were scheduled to go back to the hospital for the transfer the following day. There was a little more pep to our step the rest of that Saturday but on Sunday morning Debbie called us to cancel our transfer of the embryos.

"WHAT?" I cried. "I don't understand, you said they fertilized!" Apparently our eggs fertilized and started to divide into cells … the way that nature intended for it to happen, but then they stopped dividing. They just sat there. "Split embryos." "Delayed division," or something like that they called it. Oh my God . . . what else can go wrong? I couldn't believe it. Eli had gone to get donuts and when he came back, I gave him the foreboding news. It was written all over his face. I didn't need to say another word. We'd had it. We were done.

I couldn't stand to see my husband look like that anymore. He was emotionally exhausted from all this. No matter how bad I wanted to have our baby, it just wasn't meant to be. He would never know the joys of holding a tiny infant in his hands and looking down into sweet innocence. At least not with me. I felt guilty. I felt like a failure. I felt like I had robbed him of something so precious and beautiful. I blamed myself.

Debbie said she would call us the next day if there was any change in the situation. Yeah . . . right. We needed to face facts, face reality. It was over. That was our last shot. We were miserable all day and very surprised when Deb called us late that day and told us they would be doing the transfer after all the next day. Our little embryos may have been late in dividing but they made up the time and they were ready to go! Oh boy. Back up the roller coaster we went.

Seven days later we took the roller coaster ride back down when I started to bleed. It was over. I didn't even get to go in for the pregnancy test. That was it. All I can remember is continuous crying. Crying for all we had been through and to no avail. I would avert my eyes when I saw parents with their newborn babies or toddlers trying to get away from their moms. I couldn't stand it. Not for me . . . for Eli. I had Shannon and Buddy. I was the lucky one. I was willing to

113

gg*

share them but they weren't the babies that I wanted my husband to
hold and love.

We scheduled our post-op conference with Dr. Wayne to review the results and generally just to talk. We didn't really want to go
see him but it was part of the procedure and maybe it would give us
some closure. We reviewed all three cycles and talked about my problems with tolerating the Progesterone shots. To my utter horror, all I
could do was cry. I tried to stop but the more we talked about the three
tries, the sadder I became. Eli was angry and antagonistic. I felt sorry
for Dr. Wayne because it certainly wasn't HIS fault. We were just a
total mess. We discussed the delayed division of the embryos and discussed alternatives: adoption of course. Dr. Wayne also talked about
some new procedures they were just starting to do called: co-culture
and egg drilling. We listened half-heartedly, thanked him, shook hands
and left. On our way back to the car, Eli was already saying, "I'm glad
it's over. Let's move on with our lives. We'll lead a different kind of
lifestyle. We're going to travel and see this whole damn world."

My eyes were dry. I had new hope! I was starting to think
about co-culture and drilling eggs!

114

Chapter Eight
It'll Cost $10,000 to Put it to Bed Sir!

She Said...

So life went on. Sadly for both of us. I tried to put it behind me. I really did. But, I just couldn't let go of the thought of never having that baby. I wanted it so bad.

I threw myself into my job. Things were hectic at work. Cutbacks and layoffs forced me to put in extra long hours to compensate for the loss of people. It was the same story all over corporate America: more work, fewer people to do the work, low morale and no recognition for busting your butt. However, I truly enjoyed what I was doing. As the Manager of a Marketing Communications department, I was responsible for all the sales promotion activities, literature

generation and distribution, and trade shows and special events. There
was more than enough work to keep me busy and to keep my mind
off of the baby making process. But the corporate politics were getting out of hand. Players were changing regularly. I never knew who
my boss was going to be. During my first three years at this company,
I had nine, yes, NINE different bosses. Unbelievable. Some of the
men understood Marketing Communications, others didn't. Each one
of them wanted to make his "mark," his "statement." Consequently,
plans were continuously changing. Literature was trashed for the new
leader's "look." There was rebellion in the ranks and people were
either leaving for better pastures or trying to figure out which team to
play on in order to save their jobs.

My staff had been cut and I was buying most of the services
I needed outside. This also meant that my budget fluctuated with the
whims of whoever was currently in charge. I was never going to crack
the glass ceiling here, that was for sure. Although I believed that this
company was an excellent company to work for, if you had to work,
but this particular division was not! Poor management decisions along
with the lack of caring about the employees, had demoralized people
to the point of mutiny. I knew I would never be part of the "good old
boys network," even IF I had wanted to. It was no longer a matter of

doing a good job. It boiled down to politics and I was sick of it. 1991 was an extremely stressful year, to put it mildly. I began sending my resume out. Enough was enough. Who needed this stuff anyway?

In October of 1991, we took a New England vacation and tried to wash the stress away in the beauty of the mountains. It helped for a short time but the reality was that we had to return to the grind.

"I thought you said we were going to travel around the world?" I teased my husband.

"Yeah, we just need to win the lotto first," he'd quip back.

We were both still trying to deal with the fact that we wouldn't have a child together and consequently, were examining the age-old question . . . "Is that all there is?"

In November, Armando and Joan had their first baby; a beautiful little girl named Brittany. When we went to visit their new creation, the old pangs hit me smack square in the stomach. I wasn't jealous. On the contrary, I was so very happy for them but once again, I pitied us.

"Why can't that be us?" I cried to Eli on the way back home.

"Why can't you just put it to rest?" he angrily told me.

Every time I brought up the baby subject to my normally happy-go-lucky husband, he would shoot me down with a six-shooter.

117

He wasn't taking any chances. He argued 10 points to my one. Most of his points made sense but I still couldn't put it to rest. Something was driving me . . . something deep inside. It was more than instinct. It was as if I *just knew* that if we would try it one more time . . . we'd get lucky and have that kid! Eli refused to budge. I refused to give up.

One day we decided that it was time to trade in our car and took off for the car dealerships. I wanted a BIG car. I had always driven relatively large cars and liked the comfort and safety I felt in them. Eli wanted a Honda.

"A HONDA, are you nuts? You don't have to drive it . . . I do! What am I going to do with a Honda? They're toys!" I told him.

"Well, what kind of car do YOU want?" he asked me. "A BIG boat! How about a Cougar? How about a Buick? You know I loved my Buick LeSabre," I said.

"They're gas guzzlers. You're driving all the way to Miami every day. It'll cost a fortune in gas to drive those cars. The Honda's are beautiful now. They're practical and economical. Come on . . . you'll see," he told me.

"All right, we'll look at them, but I'm not promising anything!" I begrudgingly told him.

When my husband makes up his mind about something, there's

118

no persuading him. He usually had a valid argument about everything. He could sway the Pope to see it his way. He's persistent in his endeavors and will move heaven and earth to accomplish whatever it was he set his mind to. I often teased him about being "a dog with a bone," he just wouldn't let go until *he* was ready. Pretty much like me!

Well, he was more than determined about this. So, we went to look at the Hondas even though I had a closed mind about it and was prepared to fight if necessary!

We bought the Honda. A two-door seafoam green Honda Accord. It certainly wasn't practical for a family. I felt claustrophobic in it. I sat on top of the wheel and felt like I was driving a bumper car at a carnival. Between him and the salesperson touting the value and benefits of the car, I knew I was dead. I also knew when to pick my fights with my husband and I decided that this wasn't one that I cared enough about. He wore me down. Besides, I figured I only had to drive the damn toy for a couple of years and we'd trade again!

We celebrated our second Christmas in our new house with family and friends. We threw intimate dinner parties for six and exchanged gifts with close friends. Like an excited kid on Christmas morning, I woke up bright and early and roused my two not-so-little kids at 6:00 a.m. When they were little, they would wake me at the crack of dawn so they could see what Santa had left them. I wouldn't let them open any gifts until I had my coffee so they would have the coffee ready and waiting for me. I would wear the "Santa" hat and hand out one gift at a time so we could all "ooooo" and "awwww" together.

I still wear the Santa hat even now and hand the gifts out one at a time. Some traditions have to remain! But, I make my own coffee now and the kids don't want to get up until noon! I made them get up even though they didn't want to. I did. I remember watching my daughter and my son that Christmas morning and remembering them as little toddlers . . . ripping into their packages and squealing with joy over a new Barbie doll or a shiny red truck. As they sat beside me that day, as young adults, they opened their gifts with sleepy eyes, grumbling about being awakened so early. Oh sure, they loved their gifts but they were grown ups now. I guess I was just feeling melancholy for those precious days gone by. It's true: They grow up so fast.

As we kicked off 1992, I launched a heavy campaign to get Eli to see things my way and donate his sperm to our baby making adventure. His negative arguments frustrated the hell out of me.
"We don't have any insurance to cover it this time," he would yell at me.

"WHO CARES . . . so what? It'll come out of our savings account . . . its only money!" I would tell him as I choked on my tears.

"I don't want to go through that emotional heartbreak again . . . it's just too much to handle anymore," he told me while shaving one day.

"PLEASE . . . just one more time and then I PROMISE I'll put it to rest," I begged. No pride here.

"NO!" he stated emphatically as he threw the shaver in the sink. "Not again."

I dropped the subject until the week before my birthday in February. Sitting at the dinner table one evening I said: "You know what I want for my birthday?"

"No, but I know you're going to tell me," he said with a grin, "a new car?"

"Nope, a new baby," I said with my chin up in the air!

Dinner was a disaster that evening. Neither one of us finished eating. He got mad. I cried. Gee, for wedded bliss, I sure was crying all the time.

I didn't pursue the subject again until the first weekend in March. It was a Saturday morning and I was lying on our couch in the bedroom...waiting for Eli to finish dressing so we could go to the beach. I must have been in PMS because, once again, I just started

121

crying when I thought about the baby we weren't going to have. Eli came out of the bathroom and took one look at me and said, "Oh no, not again."

"I'm sorry. I honestly don't know what's gotten into me. Can't we just talk about this baby thing without yelling, screaming or getting angry at each other?" I asked.

"Okay, Deb, let's get it all said and move on. I can't take much more of this," he said as he sat down on the couch beside me.

I said my peace. The gist of it being: "I just know that if we try it *one more time*...we'll get pregnant. Don't ask me how I know. It's a gut feeling. It's *here* inside me. *Please, just once more?*"

As he wrapped his arms around me and held me tight he said: "All right. One more time...if that's what it's going to take for YOU to get over this...we'll do it. But, don't expect me to be enthusiastic about it."

I just smiled. And, with a bounce in my step, we drove that stupid little Honda to the beach.

We made an appointment to see Dr. David the following week but he was out of town so we would see Dr. Wayne again. That was fine with us since we wanted to talk to him about the alternatives he had discussed with us so long ago: co-culture and egg drilling. Eli needed a few answers before he would proceed. I was willing to try anything. I'd already been through the gamut more than once. There wasn't anything I was afraid of this time.

To say that Eli had an "attitude" is an understatement. He had a major chip on his shoulder. He certainly wasn't enjoying this and he seemed angry at even having to take time off from work to go to the consultation. I didn't let it deter me. We were going.

Dr. Wayne, as usual, put me at ease the moment I walked into his office. Eli was skeptical. We discussed the latest technologies that had been incorporated into IVF. Co-culture, to put it in layman's terms, is a medium in which cow fallopian tube cells are used. The cells are put into the Petrie dish, along with the fertilized embryos, in an effort to simulate the natural womb environment. All warm and cozy! We also learned about the egg drilling procedure, which is actually called: "assisted hatching." The procedure is simple. A lab technician, using a microscopic needle, simply pricks the eggshell with the needle to make the embryo hatch out of the shell easier. I thought it was fascinating; Eli remained unconvinced but willing to give it a shot. Later, we both laughed when we confided to each other that we were scared our baby wouldn't cry, it would moo!

We reviewed all of our previous cycles to pinpoint where my

weaknesses were in trying to get pregnant. While the co-culture might possibly help (everything was a gamble and there were no guarantees!) and the assisted hatching would help with slow spermies, I was still considered a "low responder." In other words, I didn't respond as well as others to the fertility drugs that I was given. However, given the three cycles we had already been through, Dr. Wayne had enough information about how I responded to different protocols to be able to devise a new protocol for us.

I had a shift in my "luteal" phase, which meant my menstrual periods weren't as regular or predictable as they had been in previous cycles. That was taken into consideration and I went back on the Ovukit to determine my ovulation cycle once again. Besides using co-culture and assisted hatching, the plan called for monitoring my FSH levels earlier in the cycle, low-dose Lupron and I would get an HCG booster...whatever the heck that meant. I would also take two injections each day consisting of a combination of Metrodin and Pergonal. This was a much higher dose than I had been previously given. It scared me a little to be taking such heavy drugs, but if the results were positive...who cared? Not me. It was a different protocol than the previous cycles so I was optimistic about it, but then I was optimistic anyway.

We started the program as agreed in late March of 1992. But, after only a few days of monitoring my FSH levels...I was canceled. Since my levels weren't where they should have been, it was not the ideal cycle to continue.

We started again in late April and after a week into the cycle, something didn't seem right to us. It wasn't that something hurt or anything like that. The protocol didn't seem right. I was doing the wrong protocol. Somehow things had gotten confused and I was on a program I had already been on in a previous cycle. I recognized that we had a problem and called Dr. David immediately. After discussing my concerns with him over the phone, I made an appointment to see him the following week. I would have preferred to just move on to the correct protocol but Eli was, to put it nicely, furious! He was just looking for any excuse to say: "See, I told you, so now can we drop it?" I was wishing that I didn't have to tell him, but of course I did.

We saw Dr. David on May 4, 1992 and he already had our file in his office, opened and waiting for us. Ut-oh! Bad news? Apparently there was a mix-up because of a new nurse and communications had broken down. It could happen to anyone, I thought. So what. Let's move on. I'm glad I recognized it before it was too late but I had every faith that the doctors would have caught it as soon as I went in for my blood drawing. Eli, of course, wanted to make a federal case out of it. He wanted someone's head and he didn't care whose it was. He would have loved to have started with Dr. David's and gone right down the line. But, thankfully, he was able to keep his temper in check and was even cordial enough to shake hands with Dr. David when we left. I wanted to hug him but I didn't. I was just glad that we were back on track.

On May 11th, we started the protocol that Dr. Wayne and Dr. David had intended for us to be on and we were off and running. A week into the shots phase, Eli had to go out of town on business again. Which, of course, meant that he couldn't administer the shots every-day. He was only going to be gone for three days but I needed some-one to shoot me up. No matter how much I wanted to, I just couldn't bear to do it myself. I considered asking Shannon to do it for me but she was just as squeamish as me about shots...so no dice there.

We thought about asking Debbie or Justine to give me my shots daily but I just couldn't manage the extra time off from work every day. My company had just had another layoff and there weren't many people left to lay off. I figured my number could be up any day so why upset the apple cart if I didn't have to. I hadn't had much luck finding another suitable position so I wasn't pressing my luck! I called

my good pal Judy again but as much as she wanted to help, it drove
her nuts the first time we solicited her and she just didn't want to do it
again.

"I know I hurt you the last time I shot you up," she told me.

"No, you didn't really," I told her as I remembered the blood she drew
every time she gave me a shot.

As the memories flooded back, I was sort of glad she declined.
Now what? We thought about asking my mother-in-law, but again the
drive was prohibitive. We finally decided to ask my sister-in-law, Marilyn, if she was willing to play nurse for me. Although she didn't think
she could really do it, Eli convinced her that she could handle it with
ease. I asked her to come spend the three days at our house so she'd
be there every morning and night to give me the shots. She reluctantly
agreed.

We invited her over one night to show her where and how to
give the injections. Eli let her practice on him...giving him "water"
shots in his arm. For those three days, she was a pro. She even began
humming when she gave me the shots. I often wondered what that
was all about. Maybe it was to calm her nerves? Whatever it was...it
worked. She only drew blood once and I barely felt the needle go into
my skin. She was almost as good as Eli. I would tease her about

127

helping to make her niece or nephew. She would roll her eyes and say, "I hope I never have to go through this." Me too. I wouldn't wish it on anyone!

On my first ultrasound visit to view my follicles, I was disappointed to learn that I only had two follicles growing. One on each ovary. I got over that quickly and looked for the positive. Two eggs... two babies. This is good.

Retrieval day finally came. June 8th. I was excited as I sat in the, now very familiar, hospital waiting room. I was a pro at this. I knew what to expect so there was no fear at all. However, I did continue to be nervous about having that IV stuck in my hand. I really detested it. I had asked Dr. David during one cycle if I could do it without "going out." No way, he informed me. End of subject. Okay...just asking.

Eli and I donned the familiar garb and took up our places in anticipation of show time. Dr. David was there along with the entire crew that we knew so well. Debbie gave me a warm blankie even though I was no longer shivering. "Just in case," she said.

I was out in minutes and awake before I knew it. I looked at my husband to find out how we did. He held up one finger. Immediately, tears formed in my eyes. He leaned down to kiss me but before he could I said: "Dr. David, only ONE egg? Are you sure?"

He gave me a little half-laugh and said: "Only one egg Deb, but it looks great. Let's hope this is our GOLDEN EGG!"

As they wheeled me into the warm and cozy room, I was thinking about what he'd said. Boy, this better be our golden egg because it's our last egg! In prior cycles, I recovered quickly and was sent home to wait for the "thumbs-up" call. But not this time. I fell back to sleep in the warm and cozy room and woke up when Eli returned from making his sperm deposit. I started moaning and groaning because SOMETHING *down there* was really hurting. It felt like something was on fire. I was still woozy and dazed from the Valium but awake enough to feel pain. Eli immediately went and got Dr. David. We surmised that it was one of my ovaries that was sore from the aspiration and Dr. David assured me that it would heal quickly and I wouldn't be in pain forever, which was the way I was feeling right then.

Nurses came in periodically to check my vitals and after a couple of hours, I was fine, awake and ready to go home. They made me stay an extra hour...just to be sure.

Dr. David called us at home that evening to make sure I was Okay.

129

"Hi, Doc, yes I'm doing fine. No problems. How's my egg?" I asked him.

"Your egg is doing fine; we'll call you tomorrow with fertilization news," he chuckled.

Debbie called us the next day and said everything was looking great. We had fertilized without any problem! So, assisted hatching may have helped here, we thought.

June 10th…another call from Debbie.

"Deb, everything looks great, we have a four-cell embryo!" She told me.

"Excellent," I said, "What time do we need to be back at the hospital?"

"Well, Dr. David has decided to wait one extra day before we do the transfer," she said. Panic set in. "WHY? What's the matter?" I wanted to know.

"Nothing, please calm down. Everything is fine. He just wants to give it a little more time to divide," she said in her most reassuring voice.

Of course, neither Eli nor I believed her. Why should we? She's not telling us something. We just knew it. Calm down, calm down. Everything is Okay. Sure.

We hardly ate or slept that evening. Eli was imagining all kinds of things.

"What if they LOST our egg?" He asked me.

"Don't be dumb, they don't lose eggs. Remember, every one's eggs are in separate containers. They can't *lose them...*can they?" I said, trying to reassure him and then starting to doubt it myself.

"What if they switch the eggs? How do we know they'll put the right egg back in you? What if we have someone else's kid?" he said in a panic tone.

"Oh my gawd...STOP IT. That's not going to happen. I'm sure they won't screw up like that. Go to sleep." I kept my fingers crossed. We didn't really sleep. We heard each other's breath and sighs all through the night.

Noon, June 11th. Debbie finally called with the news. "We're ready to transfer the embryo. Can you be here at 2:00 this afternoon?"

"No problem. We'll be there to get our baby!" I optimistically told her.

We arrived at 1:30. We were anxious. Debbie came and got us at 2:00 and took us down the hall where the transfer would be done. I changed quickly and was hanging around the room when the embryologist, came in to say hello to us and introduce himself. So here was the genius that had refined the co-culture technique. Well we sure are glad to meet YOU!

"How's our embryo?" I asked him.

"Looks great, it's now ten cells!" he proudly told us.

"WOW!" we both said in unison. We couldn't believe it had grown that quickly. So, cow cells may have helped that little egg to grow and multiply that quickly. During all of our cycles, we had never had a 10-cell embryo. This could be it, I thought to myself.

As with previous embryo transfers, this one was nice and easy. I was in the room with the VCR before I could blink. Dr. David came in to say goodbye and wish us luck.

"I'll keep my fingers crossed for you two," he told us.

"Yeah, cross everything you've got Doc...it can't hurt," I told him.

And, there I was, one last time, resigned to laying flat on my stomach for the next 24 hours, trying to eat a lobster sandwich that Eli brought me. We both were absorbed in our own thoughts while pretending to concentrate on a movie. I didn't even think about what I would do if I had to go to the bathroom. All I thought about was that they had just transferred a ten-cell embryo into me and damn it...it'd better stay in there!

Shannon brought Buddy up to the hospital that evening and we all had dinner together. When they all kissed me goodnight for the evening...I told them to say a prayer for their baby embryo!

I went home the next day in high spirits to wait the 10 days out before I could go in for a pregnancy test. On the fifth day, just before leaving for work, Eli finally broke down and said: "How do you feel... do your breasts hurt or anything?"

"No, sorry, I feel fine. I don't have any symptoms if that's what you're asking me," I said. And, of course, that's exactly what he was asking. He didn't want to get his hopes up but he had to ask anyway. I didn't want to answer him because I was afraid he'd get more depressed about the lack of pregnancy symptoms. Oh well.

He asked me again on the seventh day: "How are you feeling?" I didn't really want to answer him because I didn't want to give him any false hope but I had to tell him the truth. "Well, my nose is a bit stuffy and my boobs feel a bit swollen. Other than that, I'm fine."

I could see the light in his eyes. I was just praying that my "symptoms" weren't in my head because I wanted it so much!

When the symptoms were still there on the eighth day, he started yelling at me: "Don't pick up that laundry basket...what if you REALLY ARE PREGNANT? You'll hurt yourself, or the baby. Let me do that kind of stuff!" Oh gee, was this a taste of what was to come, IF...?

133

On the ninth day I told him I wanted to buy a home pregnancy test. He said, "NO, let's just wait." I did it anyway. I bought the test on my lunch hour and took it the minute I got home from work. It was negative. He came home and I swear he read my mind.

"You couldn't wait, huh?" he asked.

"Nope, I had to know," I said.

"And it was negative, right?" he said with an I *told* you so tone of voice.

"So what...those home pregnancy kits are a rip. They're never right. We'll see tomorrow."

We dropped the subject and tried to have a decent evening. Our nerves were raw and we needed sleep, desperately. I slept like a log that night. I was literally exhausted.

I went in for my blood test on June 22 at 8:00 a.m. The girls asked me how I felt, which translated meant: "Do you *feel* pregnant?" Fine, I told them. I refused to voice my thoughts for fear I would jinx everything. They assured me they would call me later at work with the results. I already knew!

When the call came at 3:00 that afternoon...I wasn't surprised. I was fairly calm, even though I was crying rivers of thanks. Thanking God, thanking Dr. David, Dr. Wayne, Debbie, Justine, the cow, and anyone else I could think of. I would have to go back to the office for another blood test in a few days to make sure that my BHCG levels were going up but I wasn't concerned. I was nauseated.

I sat at my desk for a few minutes, regaining my composure before I called my husband with the good news. I knew he was waiting but I needed to stop crying before I could start crying again.

"Hi honey, it's me."

"Yeah, I can recognize your voice by now did they call?" My smart ass husband asked.

"Yup...I'd love to celebrate with champagne tonight but it looks like it's going to have to be milk!" I told him.

Dead silence.

"Hon...you there?" I yelled.

"Yeah...huh? What did you say? Champagne? Oh...I get it. Oh wow." I guess he was overwhelmed. It's the first, and only time, I've ever known Eli to be absolutely speechless.

"DON'T TELL ANYONE," he was saying to me.

"WHAT? What do you mean don't tell anyone?" I said.

"I'll explain tonight. Just promise me you won't tell anyone at least until we've talked...promise me!" He begged.

"Okay. I think it's silly, but Okay I won't tell anyone. Congratulations

Dad!" I told him.

"No, Congratulations to YOU. You are something else. I'll see you tonight. Think about where you want to go to celebrate. And DON'T LIFT ANYTHING," he ordered.

I chuckled as I hung up. I would definitely find out what it was like to be a pampered pregnant wife. Boy, was I gonna love this!

We celebrated at a local Cuban restaurant…just the three of us. Shannon was so excited. She couldn't stop talking about buying baby things. She was thrilled about the baby and about being a really big sister. Over a wonderful meal and a glass of cold milk, we talked about Eli's reasons for not wanting to share the news with anyone, except family, of course. I begged him to let me tell my closest friends. He acquiesced to them but that was it. Strict orders! He was afraid that something would happen during the first three months and he didn't want anyone to know until we passed that critical marker. He also believed that negative karma, negative vibes, negative thoughts directed toward us from unknown, unnamed jealous people could result in a miscarriage. That was to be avoided at all costs. He was paranoid beyond belief but I agreed to his request even though it was gonna kill me not to tell the world. *Shhhh*…it's a secret became our motto.

We had to wait until late that night when Buddy finally came home from surfing to tell him he was going to be a big brother. When we delivered the news he said: "Hey, cool mom. Good job, dude!" We laughed. That's my Buddy.

I called Judy, Janet and Lorna the next day and they were absolutely thrilled for us.
"I knew it would happen Deb. I've never known you to go after something and not get it!"

"PREGO! That's great. You're nuts, but that's great," giggled my then single, no kids, 38 year old friend, Janet. (Little did she know that she was heading for marriage and a baby within two years herself!)

When I told Lorna, we just laughed and cried with each other! Ah, the joys of good friends!

The smiles on our faces could have lit all of Manhattan on a summer night. We couldn't have been happier. I wanted to shop. Eli wanted to wait. We argued about turning his office into the baby's nursery. He wanted to keep half the room for his office and the other half could be for the baby. He had no idea how much room babies took.

He had no idea about babies at all!

137

He Said...

I thought I had pretty much put the baby issue to bed. I had convinced myself that, for whatever reason, the man upstairs did not have children in the mix for me. I remember sitting in a lounge one night years before I had met Deb and striking up a conversation with a lady who claimed to be a fortune teller of sorts. She said she had been blessed with extra powers and that she could read palms with a very high level of accuracy. After several beers I agreed to let her read my palm, and I was truly amazed at her ability to pinpoint certain specific things about me and my past that I was sure she could not have guessed based on our brief conversation. When she finished, I remember asking her what she saw in my future with regards to children. She took my palm a second time, stared hard, and with a somewhat apologetic look she said she did not see anything in my reading associated with children. I never really gave that encounter much thought, until after our last failed attempt, and then somehow the experience crept back into my thoughts.

I was busy at work with new projects, and in order to kick-start my new life direction I even joined the company softball league. All along Deb was not at peace with herself. The topic of a fourth try came up regularly whether it was a direct statement, or the multiple subtle comments that she would drop. I wanted absolutely nothing to do with it. I was done. It was not meant to be so let's move on.

That Fall we spent ten days up in the New England area vacationing and having a wonderful time. I was so determined to reinforce the mark of our "new" life direction that on the last leg of our trip I woke up one morning and shaved off my beard. Sixteen years since my face got a breather and my bride had never seen this side of me. She stared at me for what seemed like days and all she could muster was a "WHY?" I needed a change I proclaimed, all along knowing that what I was doing was ingesting different kinds of medicine hoping that one would make the pain go away.

The holidays came and went, and I seemed to be doing pretty good until one day for no explainable reason I found myself sitting in a mall in what seemed like a trance. Anytime I was in a people-watching situation you could best bet that the ladies were a big part of the watching. Oh you know that Latin male macho stuff we all do. But this particular day was different. The mall was full of women, but I was actually staring at different men. No I had not turned the other cheek or anything like that; I was watching all the "Dads" with their kids. Playing, carrying on like kids themselves, wiping noses, holding dripping ice cream cones and stuff. For the first time since our last IVF cycle I was actually admitting to myself that maybe I wasn't really over it. That day I would have given my legs for the chance to wipe a running nose, or change a diaper full of kaka!

In February, we met with our accountant and after much discussion we decided that we needed to change the status of our corporation to a Sub Chapter S status in order to maximize our tax savings. With this change in status we would be able to combine our personal and corporate returns for maximum results. It is amazing how Deb and I think so much alike. If there is really any truth to the term soul mates then Deb and I are truly a pair. When our accountant reinforced the fact that we would be able to claim our non-reimbursable medical expenses as legitimate deductions on our return as officers of the corporation, we both looked at each other simultaneously. We both knew what the other was thinking. Deb didn't want to ask the specific question for fear that I might make a scene in the office. So I went ahead and said. "So I guess we could try IVF again and deduct the expenses off of next years return?" To this day I still do not know how those words came out of me, a certain kind of uncontrollable diarrhea of the mouth. One thing was for sure, there was no turning back. I had opened the door and there was no way I could close it. I was dead meat!

In May of that year I found myself walking down the familiar hall to the baby-making room with a cup in my hand as I had done so many times before. I was going through IVF again but this time with a different mission. I was not focusing on the possibility of having a child, but rather willing to spend $10,000 in order to help my wife bring closure to the matter. Consequently, I had a very non-chalant attitude about everything. As I opened the door to the sperm deposit room I barked down the hall to my wife in the waiting area, " I hope they finally changed the magazines in here, I'm getting tired of the same broads!"

When Dr David announced that there was only one egg during retrieval I should have retreated to the usual gloom state that this experience was so capable of creating. But there was a special kind of up beat tone in his voice when he said, "But it looks like one really nice egg." When Deb woke up and inquired as to the status of her eggs, Dr David reassured her that she had produced the "Golden Egg" this time. One egg, but it was the Golden Egg. Heck, I was starting to believe it myself! We went through the usual fertilization, embryo transfer phase without a glitch. After all we were veterans. For six weeks I had played the game, for the sake of playing. Not expecting to win, lose or draw, just play so that we could move on. But here I was counting the days until the pregnancy test results would be known. I had fallen into the trap again. I was on the roller coaster again, remembering that I had actually gotten strapped into my seat that day at Cecil's. Damn that accountant. Why was he such a good accountant after all? How dare he lead me to the carnival again, only to buy tickets to the ride again? He better know all the tax laws regarding one more dependent in the Franco family I thought…I prayed.

I had just finished getting my butt chewed by a customer on the telephone that afternoon when the phone rang again. Boy I was having a real great day, all I needed was one more irate customer telling me I ran the most incompetent department in the division and as I picked up the phone and heard my wife's voice I knew immediately that the news was good. She explained in a very poised manner that I was going to be a dad and that we were going to celebrate that night but that she had to drink milk, and the truth is I did not hear a word she said. After the initial, "Hi honey," my mind wandered as if in slow motion. I kept getting flashbacks. The palm reader, the dads at the mall, Dr David naming our egg the Golden Egg, the sterile cups, the accountant, the tears, all rolled up into one big play back. I was stunned, a happy walking zombie. I pleaded with Deb not to tell anyone for fear that we might get jinxed, and although she wanted to tell the world she agreed to

142

humor me. "Don't pick anything up sweetie, I'll do it. No groceries, no laundry, no cleaning, I'll take care of everything." Boy was I setting myself up for some torture. Oh but what sweet torture!

Chapter Nine

Keeping It A Secret . . . The First 90 Days

She Said...

I had promised to honor Eli's request about keeping our pregnancy a secret until we had passed the first critical 90 days, and then we would tell the world. Life was great! We talked constantly about the baby. Who would she (I believed it would be a girl!) look like? What color hair would she have and what would she be when she grew up? Eli was skittish about talking too much about it. He was afraid we would jinx everything if we made too many plans so I couldn't start buying things for the baby or even picking names yet. It was almost as if he was waiting for tragedy to happen. NOT ME. I felt awful and

I was so glad that I did. I didn't have morning sickness; I had afternoon sickness usually right in the middle of an important meeting at work! My co-workers, some of whom I now considered my friends, still didn't know what was going on and I was just dying to shout it to the world. But, I kept my mouth shut like a good wife. In the meantime, I was being treated like a queen. I didn't have to do anything I didn't want to do, at home that is! Eli wouldn't let me lift a thing. He didn't want me to do the laundry any more since he believed it was too heavy so he took over the job. This was great. I would do the grocery shopping on Saturday mornings and he'd be waiting for me to get home so he could bring them all into the house. If I was too tired to cook, we ate out. I have to admit that I did take advantage of that . . . I was always too tired to cook! He was so scared. Although I thought at times he was being silly, I humored him. After all . . . what did I have to lose? This was the life every woman should lead . . . pregnant or not. I was still under Dr. David's care until the end of July. He had taken two sonogram pictures of the growing fetus and in the second sonogram the baby looked like a tiny mouse. So cute. On July 30th, Dr. David advised me that I should see a specialist for an amniocentesis for genetic evaluation since I was now over 35 years of age. He also told me to contact my OB/GYN to set up my first appointment. I felt like I was being pushed out of the nest. It was so warm, comfortable and safe in his offices, I didn't really want to go, but I knew it was time. I asked him to recommend a doctor who could handle a "high-risk" pregnancy and he gave me the names of two doctors he preferred. As was customary, he would forward my records to them both. I gave him a big hug and told him I'd be in touch after we had our baby.

I decided that I wanted to talk to both doctors before I made my final decision about who would be the lucky guy! In the middle of August, I met with Dr. Eric for our initial consultation. I liked him immediately. When I sat down in his office, we had a discussion about the IVF procedure and all I had gone through. We talked about ski trips and summer vacations. I looked at the pictures of his family and checked out his certifications hanging on the wall. What I liked the most, at that time, was that Dr. Eric had already taken the time to review my file and knew everything that he needed to know about me. He didn't wait until I was sitting before him to review my file; he had actually read it and was prepared for my questions. I wanted him to be my doctor. No questions about it. I had my first exam and heard the baby's heartbeat for the first time that day. I had tears in my eyes as I listened to what sounded like horse's hooves stampeding.

I canceled the appointment with the second doctor and never

looked back.

I was still having afternoon sickness and a few times I had to excuse myself from meetings to run to the bathroom. All the time I was hugging the bowl I was wondering what my co-workers must have been thinking. First they thought I had hemorrhoids, then I had a chronic stuffy nose and cough and now I'm bolting for the door in the middle of a meeting. Weak kidneys? They must have thought I was a basket case. I made the appointment with the specialist to have my amniocentesis in mid-September. I was absolutely petrified that number one, it was going to hurt like crazy, and number two, that something would be terribly wrong and then we would have to make a decision we did not want to make. There were also risks involved, such as a possible miscarriage. That didn't sound all that great. We talked about the "what ifs" on a regular basis and I finally told Eli: "Look, number one, there's NOT going to be a problem, and number two, no matter what, I'm having this baby. End of discussion." There just weren't any alternatives for me. I had helped to make this baby, she was growing inside of me and I was going to deliver her safe and sound. Determination. Perseverance. The day arrived for the big needle to be stuck into my belly and I just couldn't stop sweating. I could feel my blood pressure rising and the palms of my hands were dripping. I also had to go to the bathroom so bad I thought I was going to wet the floor. My bladder had to be as full as possible for the amniocentesis so they encouraged me to drink as much as I possibly could. Boy, did that hurt. We were taken into a small office where a genetic counselor asked us all types of questions about our family history. She explained what the test was all about, what they would test for and told me that it was a simple, quick procedure. Easy for her to say. It wasn't her belly that was going to get a hole poked into it. At that point, I just wanted to get it over with. The anticipation and the full bladder were taking their toll on me. Let's GO!

She led us into an examination room and when I laid down flat on my back, I swore I wouldn't be able to "hold it" much longer. Eli was laughing. Yeah . . . sure, really funny honey. The doctor came in and introduced himself. Although he had a heavy mid-eastern accent and we had to struggle to understand some of what he said, he was pleasant enough and certainly efficient. I reminded him that we DID NOT want to know the sex of the baby. We wanted to be surprised. He just smiled and nodded his head. I hoped he understood me. Please don't blurt out: It's a Girl, or It's a Boy! He put some sort of clear jelly on my starting-to-protrude belly and turned on the sonogram. Together we saw the beautiful pictures of our baby. What a wonderful moment. Life truly is a miracle. She was so tiny, yet on the sonogram appeared so big. The doctor took measurements of her head and body parts and printed pictures of her that we could take home with us. She was jumping around and doing all sorts of somersaults in there and I couldn't even feel it. I wanted to feel it! Eli and I were holding hands, our eyes glued to the monitor. I wished we could have had the sonogram machine at home so we could look at her all the time. Yeah, right.

She finally settled down into one corner and the doctor gave me some anesthetic on the opposite side of my stomach. Eli just held me tight. Just as the doctor was getting ready to inject the needle, the baby moved into that exact position. Too late. We had to pick another site. The baby was in the way. The doctor explained that the baby was probably active because of all the cold water I had drunk so rather than numbing a spot again . . . let's just go for it when the baby briefly settled somewhere. And, that's what we did. OUCH! The baby settled on the left and he went to the right, stuck the needle in, withdrew the fluid and was out before she moved again. I thought I was going to faint, not from the pain but from the anticipation. It really didn't hurt that much. It was quick and over in no time. WHEW . . . done. Let's get the hell out of here.

Once again we had to wait for the results. What else was new? We were used to playing the waiting game. They told us it would be a week to ten days before we would hear anything. They would send us a letter and copy Dr. Eric. The wait was on. I prayed like I had never prayed before in my life. My mother-in-law confessed to me that she too prayed like crazy. Everyone else, the small circle of friends who knew what we were going through, kept their fingers crossed.

I came home from work one day and found the letter waiting for me. Did I dare open it without Eli being present? Of course! I breathed a sigh of relief and shed a few more tears as I read the results. Everything was fine.

She appeared to be a bit smaller than she should have been for her gestation age but she would probably catch up. I got concerned about that and started wondering if I was eating enough vegetables? Drinking enough milk? Did the kid need more protein? What? What did I need to do to make her bigger?

We celebrated our good fortune at an Italian restaurant. I gave the kid linguine with clam sauce and lots of milk. Eli drank three glasses of wine. The pressure of the amniocentesis was over and we only had two more weeks until the first trimester was over. " Breathe, honey. It's going to be okay," I told him more than once.

Eli took the sonogram pictures to work one day to show to Wayne, the only one of his friends who knew we were pregnant. Eli laughed when Wayne glanced at one of the photos and said: "Hey, the kid's got your nose." When he told me about it, I told him that was the LAST THING I wanted the baby to have of his. If dreams were to come true, I wanted the baby to have his eyes, his eyelashes and his mouth. And, the perfect kid would have my nose, my hair and my skin tone. We laughed and said the kid could look like Howdy Doody and we were going to love it! Spoken like true parents. I showed up for my second OB appointment with a grocery list of questions for Dr. Eric. I wanted to make sure I was feeding the kid right. Did I need to take more vitamins? Why was she small? And, so on. He assured me that the baby was fine. I was fine. And, yes, it was Okay to bring in my list of questions each month. That was another thing I liked about Dr. Eric. He always took the time to talk to me and answer my questions, no matter how silly or irrelevant they were. He would have a waiting room full of moms-to-be and patients behind several closed doors . . . waiting for him, but he would sit on his little stool and wait patiently while I went through my list of questions each month. I grew to not only respect and like him, but I admired him too. He had a great stool-side manner.

151

Well, we got past the first trimester without a hitch and I was starting to "show." I had a bit of a belly at the end of the third month, but by the middle of the fourth month, I had to find some bigger clothes. I started wearing stretchy shorts and Eli's shirts but it was becoming apparent that I was Prego. Eli still wanted to wait a few more weeks before letting the cat out of the bag. I wanted to buy some stylish maternity clothes and let my stomach hang out. Hell, I was proud of being pregnant and I wanted to show it off. One Saturday, I went to a local poultry market that I frequently shopped at, to get fresh chicken, fish, and produce. While placing my order with the butcher, I could feel somebody staring at me. I looked over and said: "Hi Debbie, how are you?" I had run into the wife of one of the supervisor's that worked for Eli. We chitchatted for awhile and every time I would look away, she would make a beeline for my stomach. I kept waiting for her to say something like: "I didn't know you were pregnant," or, "YOU'RE PREGNANT?" But, she never said a word to me. And, since Eli told me I still couldn't reveal my true condition, I kept my mouth shut. I could just hear the gossip at his office on Monday. I was either pregnant or I had put on some heavy duty pounds . . . right around my middle. It made me giggle. A couple of days later, I had to stop at the grocery store on my way home. As I was making my way

152

up the walkway, I ran smack into another guy, and his wife, who also worked for my husband. They were an older couple and much too polite to even stare let alone say anything. But, I knew they knew. That night, Eli and I decided to tell people as it came up. Well, it came up quickly for me. I wore a maternity dress to work the next day and it was all over the building within minutes. When the director of human resources saw me in the hall, he jokingly said: "Do you have something you want to tell us, Deb?"

"Yes, I do. I need a raise to feed an extra mouth in my family. Do you think you could arrange that?" Well, I didn't get a raise but I did get a major cold shoulder from upper management. They were not pleased that I was pregnant. Since I was in charge of all the trade shows and meetings, I had to frequently travel out of town on business. I'm sure they thought my "condition" was going to interfere with that arrangement. I was determined that it would NOT interfere with my job. So . . . we told the world! Everyone was so surprised, not that we were pregnant, but that we had undergone IVF again, without anyone knowing and that we were able to keep the pregnancy a secret for such a long time. People started asking us what we wanted . . . a girl or boy. "WHO CARES," we'd answer. "What are you going to name it?" they'd ask. "We don't know yet," Eli would say. We were in a

Chinese restaurant one night and Eli decided that we would call the baby "Pywing." We laughed at the silly nickname, but every time someone asked us about names, we would tell them with a straight face: "PYWING!"

We started making plans. I started shopping, and shopping some more. I had forgotten how much a baby required. And, there were so many new products on the market. Things that weren't available when Shannon and Buddy were babies. Did I really need all that stuff? I started making lists again. We had lists for everything. Lists for doctors, lists for baby names, lists for baby items, lists for baby doctors, lists for lists. It was getting out of control. Yet it was so much fun. One night we had a major discussion about what the odds were that a hospital could mix up your baby and you could walk out of the hospital with the wrong kid. This was a serious concern for us since the subject was a recent headline in the news. We decided the odds were in our favor that it couldn't happen to us, but how did we insure that it didn't? I begged Eli to make sure that it didn't happen by following our baby out of the delivery room and making sure they put the right bracelets on the kid and watching where they put her. "LOOK at her really well; memorize her features so you'll recognize her immediately," I told him. "Hon, all babies look alike. What good will that do?" he asked me.

"NO, all babies DO NOT look alike. Believe me. When you see your baby, you'll realize that immediately. LOOK at her. Promise me?" I pleaded. He promised me that he would follow her out of the delivery room and watch every move the nurses did with her. And, he laughingly promised to LOOK at her!

On one of my visits to Dr. Eric, I asked him for a pediatrician's name. He gave me several and once again I made appointments with two doctors who were relatively close to my home. I interviewed Dr. Paul one evening in his office. When I first met him, I thought he was too young to be a pediatrician. He was unassuming, very young looking and I just wasn't sure about him. We sat in his office and talked for about an hour. I could tell he was nervous by the way he fidgeted with his hand and kept pulling his pen out of his pocket and putting it back in there. He was probably pretty darn good with kids, but might have a problem relating to adults. Or, maybe he just needed to get to know someone before he felt comfortable. In any case, he wasn't like other doctors . . . brisk, quick, overbearing with an attitude that says: "I'm the doctor, so I know what's right."

He was called out of the office momentarily to talk with one of his nurses. There was a little boy running around the hall and I

watched Dr. Paul pat him on the head and say something to him that
made the little kid laugh. His credentials were excellent, and he had
evening, Saturday and Sunday hours to accommodate working parents.
He told me that the practice returned emergency phone calls immediately and he would always be accessible. He promised me that when
the baby was born, he would come over to the hospital to "check the
baby out." I liked him and I decided right then that he would be my
baby's pediatrician. We shook hands and departed until I would see
him at the hospital. There was still so much to do. We hadn't named
the baby yet. We bought a book of baby names to try to help us nar-
row it down. It didn't help. We still had to buy the crib, among a
zillion other things and decorate the room.

In the mean time, we started Lamaze classes. This was going
to be a natural childbirth. We went to our first class, which covered
the first trimester of pregnancy. It was boring since we were already
past that part. We were well into our second trimester, but it was fun
meeting other parents-to-be and talking about baby stuff. In one of our
classes, we talked about nutrition and my ears perked up. I was still
secretly concerned about the baby being little, even though Dr. Eric
told me that the kid was progressing nicely. We talked about cravings
and my husband told the class that I just couldn't get enough sliced

tomatoes or steak sandwiches. I was drinking alot of lemonade too. Some people had weird cravings but no one had a craving for pickles! They brought in a "baby dentist" to talk to us one night and we learned about the pros and cons of pacifiers and how to brush a child's teeth. No pacifier for our kid. A hospital administrator joined one of the classes to talk to us about hospital security and how safe our babies would be in the hospital's nursery. We talked about "baby switching" and the precautions and safety measures that were in place to insure that this horrible event would not occur. On the drive home that evening, I reminded Eli that no matter what the administrator said, I wanted him to still follow our baby to the nursery and to memorize her features! I wasn't taking any chances. In the next class we started to learn how to breathe during labor. We all felt a bit self-conscious and a little stupid doing the "hee haw" thing. Eli and I were cracking up and it became so infectious that the whole class started laughing. After that, we could practice without feeling like jerks. The instructor cautioned each husband to be patient during labor since his wife was probably not going to be her usual happy go lucky self. I knew that was an understatement. That night, the instructor went around the room asking everyone which sex their baby was and what name had been chosen. When it was our turn, Eli said: "We don't know, we

157

don't want to know, and we don't know what we'll name the unknown yet!" We were the only couple in the class who didn't know a thing about their baby! I registered for a breast-feeding class and learned that it might hurt a little in the beginning but if you were persistent, you would succeed. No problem there. Persistence was my middle name. I would be successful at breast-feeding my kid!

I also signed Eli, Shannon and myself up for an Infant CPR class. "We are all going to need to know this technique just in case," I told them. No one protested. Even if they didn't want to go, they would have, simply because I was pregnant! What power. We had to practice on a baby doll and Eli made some crack about never having had to use a blow up doll before. Men!

Chapter Ten
Nesting

He Said…

    We had survived all the hurdles of the first three months, and although I was starting to feel a little more confident that this was really happening, I still wanted to wait a little longer before we started shouting it to the world. Conversations would often come up that would lend themselves to the opportunity to tell, but each time I would bite my lip and switch gears. Deb was doing very well and right around the time she started showing she ran into people we knew who were starting to suspect that something was up. We agreed one weekend that as the opportunity came up we would start sharing our good

fortune with our closet friends. I remember calling my good friend Armando one day and asking him if he wanted to meet me for lunch. He said sure, since we had not had a chance to connect in some time.
I agreed to drive down to Coral Gables, which is close to his office. We sat for about two hours talking about everything from careers to the good ol' days, basically getting caught up. The waitress brought the check and as we were both reaching for our wallets to pay the bill and getting ready to leave I said in a very serious voice, "Armando I have something to tell you." My buddy got serious very quickly, perhaps alarmed that something might be wrong. I don't ever remember seeing him get so serious so quickly. After all, this is the same guy who used to mix Cutty Sark with Robitussin when we had our Daytona Beach escapades back in the '70's. Armando and I met and became good friends while working at an ice cream parlor called Dipper Dan. We have been friends for 20 years and although our lives are hectic and our times together are few, I still consider him my best friend. Anyway, he leaned back in his chair and said, "What's up?' I responded with, "My friend, I'm GOING TO BE A DAD!" A big smile, a warm handshake, and several congratulations later, even I felt this enormous relief. I had finally told someone! It was not easy holding back. At that point I began telling everyone as the opportunity came up. People were

great! So many of our friends knew how difficult it was for us, what an up hill struggle it had been. Now they could be part of our circle of joy. Deb was looking more and more pregnant by the day and I thought it was just great. They say women have a special glow when they are expecting. I had seen my share of pregnant women over the years, and I figured that my eyesight must have been deficient because I never detected any glow. But love is a powerful thing and it conquers all as they say including my deficient vision because I could definitely see the glow. I found her to be sexy in maternity clothes, and thought that her little watermelon sack in the nude was a real turn on. At night I would rub her belly and place my ear close trying to hear our little miracle in action. Boy was I loving this. I mean I was loving every detail, probably because I had come so close to not experiencing it, that I now felt like I couldn't miss anything.

By November I was itching to get away for a little vacation to de-stress from everything we had gone through that year. As usual I was craving cold weather so we booked a trip to Pennsylvania. I felt like taking my time getting there so I left on a Thursday morning on an Amtrak Silver Star bound for Washington D.C. I would arrive early Friday morning, and would tour D.C. that day. Deb was on a flight that would bring her in around 8:00 p.m. and I would pick her up at the airport. The next day we drove up to Amish country touring the farms and other unique attractions, lodging at cozy Bed -n- Breakfasts along the way.

On election night, as we were watching the early returns of the presidential election, and it was beginning to set in that Bill Clinton was going to lead us for the next four years, the phone rang in the room. Deb answered the phone and after a quick exchange of hellos she handed me the phone and said, "Shannon wants to speak with you," which I found kind of odd. In the spirit of not upsetting her mom, Shannon proceeded to tell me that her brother, who did not have a driver's license, had helped himself to a joy ride in our car. Unfortunately he had been involved in a fender bender with someone who was drunk, had no insurance, but who was looking to make a fast buck. I remember trying to humor myself in to restraint by replying, "Oh I see…anything important come in the mail?" After I hung up, I proceeded to rearrange the furniture in the room we were staying in, redo the walls, and basically purge my Latin temper on the surroundings. After about $2000 worth of property damage I sat down and calmly explained to my wife what had happened and that we needed to cut our trip short and get back so that we could deal with this mini crisis.

During our return flight to Ft. Lauderdale, I'm sure my wife was wondering if she was gaining one baby and possibly loosing one teenage son because here it had been 24 hours since the phone call and the subsequent tirade and I was still blurting out four letter expletives. Boy was I mad!

By late January the crisis had passed, the holidays had been great, with much talk about how the following Christmas would be with the baby around. We had bought alot of baby stuff including the crib, dresser and changing table set. I am not the Bob Villa type so I had to pick a day that I was in the right frame of mind to assemble the furniture. One night during the week, after hearing enough of the "When are you going to assemble the furniture?" I decided to take on the project. I solicited Shannon's assistance while Deb read the directions. Piece by piece we were putting the set together. We finished around 2:00 a.m. totally exhausted, but excited because it was just one more affirmation that this miracle was really happening. I swear I pinched myself continuously, waiting to wake up from this beautiful dream.

The third Sunday of the month was a special day. My wife was having her baby shower, but what was really special was that it was her daughter who was throwing the party for her. Now that wasn't too common, but then again everything about us is sort of atypical. I was

163

politely thrown out of the house for the day; not being allowed anywhere near the day's festivities. This was absolutely fine with me. I spent the day at the beach soaking in the winter sunshine, basking in the virtues of anticipated fatherhood. It was a great day all around. The Miami Dolphins lost in the playoffs, which really made it a great day since I am a loyal Minnesota Vikings fan. I came home to find tons more baby stuff all over the house, chocolate layered cake, and a video that captured some precious moments in Debbie's life. Boy I just could not imagine life getting any better. Our baby's target date was early March and we were in the stretch run now, a few more weeks, a few more loose ends to tie, and we were ready for show time.

Everything was going right along, just like we had mapped it out in the game plan.

Or so we thought!

Chapter Eleven
The Phone Call

He Said...

Charlie was not easy to get close to. He was an astute business manager with a dry sense of humor and unparalleled wit. I learned alot of different things from Charlie. Patience, the art of "holding off" until the absolute right moment. Understanding all of the resources available, sizing up the big picture. I felt that I had matured under Charlie, and was very appreciative of the opportunity to work under and for the man. By the same token Charlie and I did not always see eye to eye. I had the utmost respect for Charlie, and I felt that he respected my ability to manage. After all the man promoted me to department head status with a group of 90 employees to supervise at the tender age of 24. With a certain confidence and youthful cockiness, I would from time to time vehemently argue my point of view with Charlie about a variety of business issues. Sometimes we did it his way. Sometimes we did it my way but I always found a way to make sure he was secure in feeling that it was his final ruling.

For the past 15 months Charlie and I had been at odds about cellular phones. I felt that in my position, with the amount of time in the field and the frequency with which I was being paged for some type of emergency, that a cellular phone was a necessary working tool in order to work smart. Charlie felt that it was more of a toy than a necessity. And so, we sparred continuously, sometimes to the point where I felt that if I opened my mouth one more time I was going to get canned. Finally, with Wayne's support we were able to get Charlie to acquiesce. I felt great the day two of my colleagues, Rafael and Jesus, and I got our car phones installed in our company cars. I think we called each other for two hours just to try out all the features. As much as I lobbied for car phones because of the need to conduct business, ironically one of the first calls I received on my new phone was very personal in nature. It was about six in the evening and I was already on my way home when the phone rang. When I answered it was Deb

166

on the other line calling me in somewhat of a panic. "I just left Dr Eric's office and he says that he needs to admit me to the hospital immediately." "What's wrong?" I muttered barely catching my breath from the sudden surge of panic. "He says my blood pressure is very high, and it could pose some risks to the baby." "Okay, we'll talk as soon as I get home." Now, not only was I guilty of using the phone for personal use, I was about to break all of the Smith System Driving techniques I had learned the week before. If that Ford Tempo could have done 100 mph I would have.

By 7:30 that evening Deb was in a bed in the Critical Care Unit of Hollywood Memorial Hospital with multiple monitors strapped to various parts of her body. A team of doctors, nurses, technicians, assistants and just about anyone else who happened to be around, were monitoring pressures, temperatures, heartbeats, breathing and all sorts of other vitals. After a series of tests the decision was made to keep Deb in the hospital overnight for observation. Of primary concern was to get her blood pressure under control for her well being as well as the baby's. I would get my first lesson on fetal monitoring, and a condition called pre-eclampsia. Another doctor was called in who specialized in treating this condition and as it turned out he eventually became Deb's cardiologist. Deb spent the next two days in the hospital, complaining all along that she was fine and that she wanted to go home. By now her employer was notified that Deb was going out on leave because of complications. I had felt all along that Deb had waited too long to go out on leave, but she kept insisting that she felt well enough to work and carry her normal load. While this was going on, Vice Presidents from corporate were coming in and out of the division meeting with the various managers. One in particular was in my office one morning conducting an intense meeting with me behind closed doors. Unbeknown to us at the time, Charlie had already let the President of our company know that he was retiring at the end of the year. I guess corporate was still undecided as to whether Wayne was going to be given the Division Manager's job, so we were getting alot of visits from the brass. So in the middle of this very important meeting my phone rang and of course I answered it. Deb was venting her frustration because she still did not have a definitive answer as to when she could go home. So here I was, with this VP in my office trying to get to know me a little better, and I am saying things like, "Hang in there honey; it's going to be all right sweetie." Luckily he was more than understanding, and in retrospect I do not believe that it cost me points on the corporate vine.

We finally went home, but with new ground rules. Certain diet changes, complete bed rest, certain new medications, and a constant vigil on Deb's blood pressure. We were given a portable blood pressure machine so that we could monitor her pressure every 4 hours. Naturally the first machine they gave us was defective which caused us to go into a frenzy one night as we were trying to assess Deb's condition. All along we were focused on the baby's movement or general level of activity. Some days the baby was active and we felt great. Other days the baby did not move much and we worried sick. We actually had a goal. We needed to get past week 38 so that the baby's lungs would be fully developed. Full gestation was 40 weeks. We were almost at week 35. We needed to hang on another three weeks.

During the next two weeks we were in and out of the hospital, first, on an out patient basis for regular testing and fetal monitoring. At one point Deb was readmitted for another two-day stay because they thought things were not going well. Then they sent her home again, and we resumed our out patient routine. Ah ha! A new roller coaster. All along things had gone perfect, but now so close to the finish line we were in for our final ride. I had been so upbeat, so positive about the whole experience up to this point. But now I was beginning to have my doubts. The reality was that I was not a dad yet. Maybe I had taken too much for granted. Oh no, the fortune tellers face started haunting me again. Maybe she was right after all. Maybe children just weren't in the cards for me. I just could not believe that this was happening to us at this stage in the game. We had endured so much in the last three years. Four IVF attempts, the amino, eight months of picture perfect pregnancy, how could things get screwed up now, I asked myself.

I remember drifting back to the day when we finally picked our names for the baby. We had procrastinated till the end. After months of searching through baby name books we finally decided on Madison if it was a girl. It was different, not at all common and full of character. Madison Elizabeth Franco. I could see her in a blue pinstriped suit, making her closing arguments in the courtroom. My daughter the successful trial lawyer. How did we miss kindergarten, puberty, and high school graduation? Picking a boy's name was even more time consuming. There must have been some little voice inside that kept saying don't sweat it bub, no need to pick out a boy's name. About a week before this whole ordeal we were sitting in our doctor's office when I picked up another baby names book, and there it was. Ellison, son of Elias. Plain as day. And so we decided on Ellison James Franco.

After snapping out of my momentary daydream, I was back in the real world, wondering what destiny had up its sleeve.

Chapter Twelve

Don't Pack . . . We'll be Back Home by Late Morning!

She Said...

We were scheduled for another fetal monitor test on February 5th at 9:00 a.m. Eli took me to the hospital where a nurse hooked me up to the monitor machine. We could hear the baby's heartbeat but there was very little movement. Come on kid, move, I thought.

After nearly 30 minutes without much activity going on, the nurse brought me a cold glass of water to drink. That should wake the kid up. The water made the baby wake up but no significant activity was noticed.

A phone call was made to Dr. Eric to report the results and to keep him current on our situation. He told them to keep me on the monitor for another hour and then to call back. After an hour of sitting in the chair, listening to the heartbeat but not getting the kind of movement we expected, the nurse called Dr. Eric again.

Dr. Eric ordered a sonogram and after awhile I was put into a wheel chair and taken upstairs to the sonogram area. I waited there for what seemed to be forever before I had my sonogram. The technician confirmed that the baby had not turned yet…the kid was still breech. I didn't know what else they were looking for but it was a long sonogram and she made quite a few notes. I asked questions but I apparently either wasn't asking the right ones, or I wasn't getting the answers I wanted. I was starting to worry and didn't know what I was supposed to be worried about. Was my baby okay?

The sonogram people were finished and I was wheeled back downstairs to the testing area where they put me back on the fetal monitor and encouraged me to eat some lunch. No thanks. I'm not hungry.

Eli called Wayne to let him know what was going on and to tell him that he might not be into the office until later in the afternoon. He looked so worried and haggard. I wasn't hungry but told him I was starving so he would leave and get us some lunch. He needed a break.

While Eli was gone, I sat in the chair reading a magazine, wishing I could go home. What the heck were we waiting for? I finally cornered a nurse and asked her when I would be able to go home? She told me that they were waiting for the sonogram results to fax over to Dr. Eric and then she'd let me know. Oh. Okay. I waited.

When Eli returned, I told him we were still waiting and he was starting to get mad. Enough was enough. His patience was again running thin. He either wanted to have a baby or go to work. Cut and dry. We had just about made the 37 weeks mark and I didn't know how much more stress we could take. We ate our lunch and waited for some news. The baby liked her lunch because she woke up and started moving a little bit. I started to have a few cramps and wondered if I was going into labor. When the nurses checked the printout from the monitor, they could see that the baby had moved somewhat but she still wasn't her usual active self. They also asked me if I was feeling labor pains. I told them I was crampy but not in pain.

Everything was reported back to Dr. Eric. Around 3:00 p.m. a chipper nurse came in to tell us that Dr. Eric had decided to induce labor. Perhaps a few labor pains would entice the baby to turn into the correct position for birth. Eli was ecstatic. He stood up immediately and started heading for the door.

173

"Where are YOU going?" I asked him.

"I don't know, I'm just getting ready. It's show time!"

I wasn't so thrilled. I wanted to go home. I was supposed to have the-baby at Memorial WEST, the NEW hospital . . . the one we had toured. Not Memorial EAST . . . the OLD hospital. Ah, man, we hadn't even finished our Lamaze classes! How was Eli going to know what to do? It didn't look like I had any choice in the matter and we were just going to have to wing it. I took a big breath and tried to steady myself for the upcoming event.

We were taken upstairs to the maternity wing and led into a birthing suite similar to those at Memorial West. At least that was comforting, I thought. I was given a gown to change into and then was hooked up to another monitor and an IV was started. Although I was apprehensive, I wasn't too scared since I had been down this road twice before. I basically knew what to expect and I figured this kid would turn around and pop right out.

I went through minor labor pains for about an hour. I hardly felt them, just some heavy cramping. Hey, I can certainly handle this. No problem. The nurses could monitor my pains for degrees of intensity so they knew I wasn't feeling too awful much. Eli and I were both excited that we were finally going to have our baby, but apprehensive that everything would turn out all right. Eli was stuffing chewing gum into his mouth like it was going out of style. I was laughing at him because he was acting like the typical nervous husband, soon to be father. He left me for a brief time to run to the phone and call Shannon at work to let her know that her baby brother or sister was on the way. When he returned, Dr. Edward, one of Dr. Eric's partners, was in the room with me. It was now 4:30 in the afternoon and we had been at the hospital all day. Dr. Edward told us that he wanted to do an internal exam to see if the baby had turned yet. Any woman who has ever had an internal exam at this stage of the game knows what horrible pain that is. When he was done, he told us that the baby had not turned yet and he was going to consult with Dr. Eric. Fine, I thought. Where the hell was Dr. Eric anyway? I had only met Dr. Edward once in the office and I really didn't want him there. I wanted Dr. Eric! When I asked the nurse what HE was doing here she told me that he was on call for the evening so he would probably be delivering my baby.

"OH NO," I told her. "We've been in contact with Dr. Eric all day long. He knows me, he knows what I've been through, he's been my doctor for seven months and just because Dr. Edward is on call is no reason for him to flake out on me now. I really want Dr. Eric here!"

I was calm, cool and insistent. Things were not going as planned and the last thing I wanted to deal with was a strange doctor. It was only 5:00 p.m. Surely Dr. Eric wasn't "off-duty" at 5:00 p.m. Eli was telling me to chill out, relax. He didn't understand the patient/doctor relationship one builds with their OB!

The nurse left the room and Dr. Edward. returned and informed us that they were going to do a Cesarean section.

"You have got to be kidding," I said half jokingly and half seriously. "This is not the way this is supposed to be going. What happened to inducing labor and seeing if the baby turns?" I cried.

Dr. Edward. explained that the baby had not turned at all and that it didn't seem likely that it was going to happen. "Can't I just go home and wait for the kid to turn?" I implored.

"No," he said patting my hand, "we need to do the C-section."

When he left the room I grabbed Eli's hand and in one breath said: "Tell me everything you've read about C-sections . . . quick!" Eli laughed and said, "Everything's going to be fine sweetie . . . stop worrying." Oh sure, easy for him to say. He wasn't the one that was going to have his belly sliced open shortly. Give me labor pains!

I basically knew what a C-section was all about but the anticipation was nerve racking. A few minutes later a whole army of nurses converged on me. Prep this. Shave that. Needles here. My blood pressure skyrocketed. I was sweating beyond belief. The sheets were off of my private parts and lights were shining down there. An automatic blood pressure cup was attached to my left arm and when it registered a reading, the nurse who was shaving me looked up and with bulging eyes said: "Geez, look at her blood pressure . . . give her something!" I looked at Eli in panic. Was I going to die?

The nurses did their thing in 15 minutes or less. The anesthesiologist was next. This big hulk of a man with coke rim glasses came into the room to insert my epidural. We never got to go to the epidural class either but I had read enough about the procedure and figured this couldn't be any worse than what I had already been through. Let's get it over with.

One of the nurses came back into the room to help with the procedure. I was told to sit on the edge of the bed and arch my back like a cat. It was easier to do this with my arms around the nurse's neck. She was great. She kept whispering silly things to me to help me calm down and periodically reminded me to keep my back arched. I could feel the adrenaline rushing through my body. The anesthesiologist was having a hard time inserting the tube, and he told us about it.

He took a big breath and let out a loud sigh and said: "This darn thing just doesn't want to go in." I looked at Eli, begging him to do something, anything, but he was powerless. This guy was scaring the hell out of me. "I have tickets to the game tonight and I don't want to be late. Why won't this go in?" he yelled with exasperation. "I'm not even supposed to be here right now, but the next shift is late getting here!" he shouted. Eli told him, "Hey, calm down man, you'll make the game."

Don't take it out on me, I thought. What the heck did I ever do to you? I looked up with frightened eyes at my Florence Nightingale and said: "I'm seeing black spots in front of my eyes." Eli was pacing and chewing gum so fast I thought he was going to break his teeth.

After the third try, the hulk finally got the epidural in and immediately administered anti-blood pressure medicine to bring my pressure back down. Thanks for nothing, jerk. Go to your stupid game. Get the hell out of here. He left without a backward glance at me.

At 6:00 p.m. the door to my room opened and in walked Dr. Eric. I was so glad to see him I started to cry but immediately found myself calming down.

"Hi, how are you doing?" he asked. "You don't want to know," I told him. I wasn't about to relay the epidural horror to him. Not now

178

anyway. He checked me out, assured me everything was going to be fine and then told me that Dr. Edward. would be doing the C-section. He would be assisting. Fine with me, as long as he was there . . . I felt safe and secure. He pinched my belly and asked if I could feel it. I felt a little pressure but that was it. We were ready but apparently we were waiting for the anesthesiologist.

The next thing I knew, Shannon and Buddy were walking into the room. Shannon had the camera and the video camera with her to record the momentous occasion. *No, don't take pictures of me, I look awful.* The truth was that my makeup, down to my lipstick, was all still perfectly in place. Incredible. But, before I could protest, Dr. Eric was posing on one side of the bed, Eli was on the other and she was snapping away. Unbelievable, but true.

"Enough you guys. Out. We'll see you in a little bit...as soon as I get this baby out of me!"

I sent them both packing. I found out later that they both wound up sitting on the floor outside the family waiting area because there weren't any chairs in the room. Apparently a woman with a huge family was giving birth next door to me and the whole family turned out for the event. Dr. Eric was losing his patience and asked the nurse where the anesthesiologist was . . . we needed to get going. "NOW," he told her as he left the room. Within minutes I was wheeled into the surgery room to deliver the baby. Dr. Edward , Dr. Eric, my Florence Nightingale nurse and a host of other people were in there waiting for me. As they picked me up and transferred me to the operating table I was thinking oh my gosh, I must weigh a ton; how embarrassing! I'm going to go on a diet as soon as I'm done breast-feeding.

I heard Eli saying, "I thought you had a game to go to?"

I turned my head and saw the hulk anesthesiologist. OH NO. NOT HIM AGAIN.

"Yeah, the other team should be here shortly," he said in a soft tone.

"OK, Deb, we're going to begin. Just relax." Yeah, sure . . . with the hulk here.

Eli and I were holding hands and smiling at each other. I felt a tap on my right shoulder and a young man asked me how I was doing. It wasn't the hulk! Apparently the second shift guy arrived and the hulk left before I knew it. GOOD.

"I'm doing great now," I told him. I wonder if he thought I was flirting with him. Imagine, a woman in my condition!

"Eli, do you want to stand up and watch now?" Dr. Eric asked

Eli stood up but didn't let go of my hand. "Tell me what you see Hon," I yelled. He didn't speak. He was chewing his gum so hard and so fast that all of a sudden he broke a cap on one of his teeth. It went flying across the room and one of the technicians in the room picked it up and gave it back to him. It all happened so fast that we didn't even have time to react to it. Dr. Eric was saying: "IT'S A GIRL!"

"Ah . . . a girl . . . I knew it!" I cried, tears flowing freely. Eli was hugging and kissing me and we both were letting those emotions loose. We had done it. We had a baby girl. Madison Elizabeth Franco entered this world on February 5th, 1993 at 6:24 p.m.

A nurse had the baby and brought her over to me briefly so I could see her. She was screaming her guts out. Oh, she's so tiny. I watched them weigh her; 4 pounds, 1 ounce. A preemie. Eli was over on the other side of the room with the baby, watching everything they were doing . . . just like he was supposed to be doing.
"Is she all right?" I yelled over to him. "Does she have everything?" He was shaking his head yes, yes, yes. He couldn't talk. Emotions. The nurses were cleaning her and doing all sorts of things to her and as I watched I started becoming aware of PAIN. Oh, I hurt. I started to moan and Eli came over to me just as Dr. Edward said: "Why is she moaning . . . what's going on?" They gave me more drugs and I didn't feel a thing as he started his re-patching job.

Once Eli saw that I was calm again, he went back over to the baby. They had her in an incubator and were starting to wheel her out of the surgical area. Eli was following close behind.

"No, no don't leave me," I screamed to him.

"Don't leave me alone."

"Hon . . . you told me to follow her . . . what's the matter?" I had no idea what the problem was; I just didn't want him to leave me. He sat down and took my hand and that's all I remember. I was out. I woke up in the recovery room. Eli was sitting next to me with a worried look on his face.

"What's the matter? Is the baby okay?"

"Yeah, as far as I know," he said, "They're checking her out, she's in the intensive care neonatal unit."

"Oh no." And, of course, I started crying.

Shannon and Buddy showed up shortly after that and I tried to put on a brave face for their sake. They were so excited. We kissed and hugged and cried together. They had been burning up the phone lines . . . calling everyone with the good news. I told them to go home and get some rest. I needed the rest. I told Eli to go home too, but of course, he wasn't going anywhere. Shannon took Buddy home but returned within an hour. I kept dozing and waking up. I wasn't feeling too much pain and I had a false sense of security that this was going to be a breeze. C-sections weren't that bad after all. Shannon came into the recovery room with her friend, Hala, carrying balloons and stuffed animals. It was so very sweet of them, but I was so very exhausted. I just wanted to sleep. Eli would leave when I slept so he could make phone calls and grab a bite to eat. Finally, around 9:30 that evening I insisted that they please go home, I really wanted to sleep. They finally left me alone and went home. At 11:30 that night, I was coming out of that fuzzy anesthesia stage and the nurses said they would be taking me up to my room then. Good . . . but first . . . where the heck was my baby? They said they would try to see if they could take me into the neonatal unit before they took me up to my room. Okay, I'm ready, let's go. I got to hold my baby for the first time just before midnight. Tears rolled down my cheeks as I was kissing her and checking her out to make sure all of her was there. The nurses took a few Polaroid pictures of the baby and me and gave them to me so I could have them in my room. She was so tiny and I was so worried. They told me she was a "healthy preemie." I had no idea what that meant. I was told the doctors would talk to me in the morning. I reluctantly gave my baby back to them and let them take me to my room. I felt so guilty about her being a tiny preemie. Did I do something wrong? What happened? I swear I drank milk, took my vitamins, and did everything Dr. Eric told me to do. PLEASE LET HER BE OKAY.

PLEASE, I prayed like I had never prayed before.

Chapter Thirteen
Our Little Preemie

She Said...

The next morning I woke up feeling like pure dog meat. Although I still wasn't in any unbearable pain, I felt like I had been run over by a Mac truck. I was exhausted, mentally and physically. "How is my baby? Is she Okay? When can I see her?" I bombarded the first nurse who crossed my path. "Everything is fine, the doctor will be up soon," I was told.

The nurse helped me get out of bed to sit in a chair. Bad move! Yesterday's lunch was no longer. I was sitting in the chair when the neonatal unit doctor arrived. He told me that Madison was doing fine, she was jaundiced and had some problem with her blood cell count. I had no idea what the heck he was talking about. He didn't spend too much time with me since he could see I was in no shape to talk right then. I figured my pediatrician would be there that morning to examine her and he would give me the straight scoop. I called Eli and asked him to bring the bag that I had packed for the hospital but to first stop in and see how the baby was doing. Like I really needed to ask him to do that! Silly me. I laid back down in the bed and wondered if my baby was going home with me. As I was lying there, the right side of my face started to feel funny. It was getting numb. I thought that maybe this was a side effect of the anesthesia, or perhaps a side effect of the epidural. Within minutes the entire right side of my face was totally numb. It was frozen solid. I grabbed the side tray and looked inside for a mirror. When I saw my face, I panicked. What was going on? I couldn't smile. My eye was frozen, my cheek was frozen, and half of my lips were frozen. I was lopsided. I looked like a geek, a gimp. And to top it all off, I was starting to feel some serious pain from my incision. I frantically rang the bell for a nurse. When she came in to see me, I didn't need to say much for her to see that something was terribly wrong. She told me Dr. Eric was on his way over for morning rounds and she would have him see me immediately.

"Dr. Eric . . . look at me . . . what is this?" I cried while pointing to my frozen face.

He examined me and said it might be, could be, a Bell's Palsy. A temporary form of paralysis. WHAT? This couldn't be happening! My baby was downstairs somewhere…fighting for her life, and I was stuck up on some numberless floor, helpless, in pain. I couldn't get to her…and now they were telling me I was paralyzed? This was not in the script! More tears.

Dr. Eric ordered a pain medication and told me he would call a neurologist to come and see me that morning. Eli arrived and reported on Madison's condition. "She looks fine," he told me. He looked awful.

"They've taken tons of blood tests and other tests and she has no lung problems. She does have a low white blood cell count but that should get under control shortly," he continued in a monotone voice.

"And she's jaundiced. She's got a blindfold over her eyes and they've got the bilirubin lights on her. But, they told me that she's a healthy preemie," he said as he tried to smile.

Before I could ask what they meant by a "healthy preemie," he took one long look at me and said in a desperate voice: "What the hell is wrong with your face?" "Oh nothing, I'm just paralyzed. How do you like being married to a gimp?" I tried for humor, unsuccessfully.

I explained what Dr. Eric had told me and as I was finishing my story of woe the neurologist arrived. He put me through a series of eye/hand coordination moves and other tests and declared that it indeed was a Bell's Palsy, not a stroke, and it would resolve itself on its own. Well, thank goodness for that, "How long do I get to look like Popeye?" I asked him. He laughed and said it could take any-where from four weeks to a year to clear up. Great. There wasn't any medicine I could take to make it go away sooner. I had to drink out of a straw and chew on my left side.

I learned how handicapped people felt when others stared at them, or snickered, or made snide remarks. It was embarrassing, degrading and a total nuisance. But, it could have been worse. It could have been a stroke and I could never have recovered from it. I had something to be grateful for. I never did find out what caused the Bell's Palsy but Eli and I suspect that it was caused from extremely high blood pressure . . . like when I was seeing black spots before my eyes. We moved on. We had more pressing things to worry about . . . our preemie baby. The only way I could see the baby was if someone took me down to the neonatal unit in a wheel chair. When the special-ist left, I asked Eli to take me down there so I could see her. When we got there, I took one look and started to bawl like a baby. What a sight I must have been with only half of my face crying. Gross. Madison had a tiny little diaper on that didn't fit her and she was lying on her side. She had blinders on her eyes to prevent any damage while she was under the lights to treat her jaundice. An IV was sticking out of her little head and I could see marks all over her tiny feet where she had been pricked for blood samples. My poor little baby. I could barely stand up so I couldn't really reach into her incubator to touch her. Eli and I held each other and said she was beautiful!

He took me back upstairs to my room where a nurse was waiting to give me a sponge bath. I was just getting ready to do that when my in-laws appeared. I really didn't want any company and didn't want anyone to see me in my Palsy condition. I could barely walk, let alone talk and my emotions were hanging out for anyone to see. "I know you want to see the baby so please go see her and come back later," I told them.

When they didn't return, I was afraid I had hurt their feelings, but Eli assured me that they understood. Shannon showed up after I had the bath and another dose of pain killers so I was feeling better. She would have stayed all day but the nurses kicked her out and told her I needed to rest. I did. I was tired. I slept for four hours straight and woke up to a room full of flowers and balloons. The phone was ringing, the word was out. Yes, I'm fine. I explained about the baby. I didn't talk about the Palsy. Vanity.

Eli, Shannon, Buddy and I all visited the baby that evening. She wasn't under the lights and had her eyes open. But, she still had the IV in her head and we could only touch her through the opening in her incubator. You could see the worry on the kid's faces. I put on false bravado. Everything was going to be fine.

The next morning Dr. Eric removed my stitches and told me he was going to keep me in the hospital one more day because they were still concerned about my blood pressure. It was fluctuating regularly and medication was necessary to keep it in normal limits. Fine with me. I could stay close to my baby. I was starting to walk a bit better. Practice makes perfect.

I was already in the wheel chair, holding a little stuffed bunny to bring to Madison, when Eli came that morning. I wanted to see my baby. I wanted to bond with her. He wheeled me down stairs and when we walked into the unit, our baby wasn't where we had left her. We looked at each other in horror. Where was our kid? You could hear the beating of our hearts. One of the nurses saw the terror on our faces and came rushing over.

"Madison graduated to the next unit," she said with a huge smile on her face.

"She doesn't need intensive care, we put her over into the 'well-baby' neonatal unit," she told us.

Big, huge sighs of relief escaped from both of us. The second level neonatal unit was just across the hall. Eli wheeled me in there and we searched for our kid. We zeroed in on her immediately. Proof positive that all kids do not look alike! She was doing better. She wasn't out of the incubator yet, and she still had the IV, but I could hold her. I fed her a bottle and put her on my shoulder so she could nuzzle up under my ear. Eli held her with awe. He liked to hold her with her head in his palm so he could look at her face. She would stare right back up at him. We learned to read the doctor's charts. We knew what her temperature and her weight were at any given hour. We asked about her feeding schedule so we could be there for that special time. She would cry when we put her back into her little bassinet, as if she knew we were leaving her again.

On the third day, I started getting horrific headaches. Real pounders. Now what? Dr. Eric ordered medication for the headaches. I was pumping breast milk into tiny doll-size bottles to bring downstairs to Madison every day. I was afraid all the pain medicine was going to have an adverse effect on either my milk or my baby. I was assured that neither would happen. I got impatient waiting for Eli to get to the hospital so I got in my wheel chair and took myself down stairs to see my baby. It took me awhile to get there, but I was a determined mom! Eli would find me sitting by the incubator and together we would spend that precious time holding her, kissing her, loving her and most important, bonding.

The next day, I had to leave the hospital without her. I hated it. They wheeled me out with 10 baskets of flowers and balloons that said: It's a Girl. But no baby girl was in my arms. I stopped in the unit to say goodbye to her and my heart wrenched to leave her there. Eli had to drag me away. When we arrived home, I saw a huge banner hung on the front door, announcing the arrival of the miracle baby. Shannon had hung the banner on the day the baby was born and I left it hanging until after I brought her home. I wanted her to see it too!

That night, our friends, Rebeca and Rafa, came knocking on the door and delivered a feast fit for a king and queen. They wouldn't even come in the front door because they knew I wasn't feeling up to company. With huge smiles on their faces they just gave me the homemade, scrumptious meal along with a few hugs and kisses and said: "We'll see you when you're feeling better," and they were gone!

Of course, I cried and realized how lucky we were to have so many people who cared about us and loved us.

We fell into a routine dictated by Madison. Eli would go to work in the morning and I would call the hospital after her morning feeding to see how she was. She had good days and bad days. Some days she was progressing well, keeping her milk down, and wetting her diapers. They took the IV out of her head. Finally. Other days, she couldn't keep anything in her tummy, she would run a fever, lose a few ounces, or she'd get constipated. They put the IV in her foot. We were on another roller coaster ride. She needed to weigh 5 pounds before we could take her home. I would call the hospital every few hours to check on her. I'm sure the nurses were getting sick of hearing my voice on the other end of the phone, but I could have cared less. When Eli got home from work, we would head straight to her. We had a ritual when we arrived.

* Wash hands.

* Put breast milk in refrigerator and get empty bottles for the next days milk supply.

*Talk to nurse to get condition update.

* Pick Madison up and hold her for as long as we could.

* Nurse would weigh her and take her vitals.

* Give Madison sponge bath and change her into clean PJs for the night.

* Feed Madison her bottle.

* Sing lullabies and rock Madison to sleep.

She was finally out of the incubator and in a tiny bassinet. We could touch her and hold her all we wanted. As tiny as the bassinet was, she was still just a tiny little ball curled up in it. There were other babies in the unit who filled the bassinet and I wondered why they were in there. I found out that some of them had internal problems and required surgery. Poor little things. Poor parents. I knew we were the lucky ones. We discovered the meaning of "healthy preemie!"

The weighing part of her routine became critical. The hospital recorded the weight in ounces, which we quickly converted to pounds. Every ounce was a milestone. Her bottle held two ounces of breast milk and we were jubilant when she finally drank all two ounces of it. "Good girl!" we would tell her, over and over. We both wanted to do it, so we took turns feeding and bathing her. One of us would feed her while the other took video so we could record the memories. We took miles of video.

Once I was able to drive again, I would spend the day at the hospital. We bonded well. She was recognizing the sound of my voice. I tried to breast feed her . . . she wanted nothing to do with it. She was already used to the bottle so I just kept pumping to give her the breast milk anyway.

After 3 ½ weeks, she finally hit the 5-pound mark. We were told we could take her home the next morning. YEAH!

We arrived with a car seat in hand, another new jammie for her to wear home, and smiles illuminating our faces. We were taking our miracle baby home. I was just picking her up when the nurse came over and said the doctor wanted to talk with us. What? What does he want? Didn't we pay our bill? Are they going to hold our kid ransom? The doctor felt that he shouldn't release her yet since she had run a small fever the night before. He wanted to keep her a little longer for observation. We were devastated. What for?
Come on!

Although she wasn't currently running a fever, it didn't matter. He wanted to make sure she wasn't going to run one again. Dejected, we had to leave without her. Eli had an appointment with our accountant that afternoon so we had to go home so I could get my car and go back to the hospital by myself. We kissed her goodbye and left.

The phone was ringing off the hook when we got home. "Mrs. Franco, this is Memorial Hospital calling," said a crisp, clear female voice.

Oh no, something happened to my baby. Well, apparently after group consultation, the hospital had decided to release Madison after all since she would be released to the care of her private pediatrician. Hallelu-jah!!!!

"Eli, let's go get her," I cried excitedly. "Deb, I've got that appointment let's wait until after that to get her," he told me, "We'll pick her up around 6:00 p.m."

"No way, I want my baby, I'll go get her myself then, I want her home," I insisted. I was afraid the hospital doctors would change their minds. I didn't want to take any chances. He went with me, of course.

We dressed that little baby so fast and put her into her car seat to take her out of the hospital. She was dwarfed in the car seat and she screamed her guts out when I put her in there and strapped her down.

Scream all you want kiddo, you're going home!

He Said...

I woke up capless the next morning but with a new title to add to my personal resume: DAD. I went over to my parent's house early to walk them through what had happened the day before in more detail since I really did not get into it over the phone the evening before. We agreed to meet at the hospital later that morning so that they could meet their granddaughter. When I arrived at the hospital I stopped in to see Madison first. She was wired up with various monitors; an IV married to her scalp, and feet that looked like pincushions from all the blood testing. I was happy and sad at the same time because I really was not in a position to enjoy the miracle of birth. My daughter was hardly out of the woods yet, and then things compounded when I went upstairs to see Deb and found out that she had paralysis of the face. Boy, when do I start having fun I asked myself. Most dads are shooting video and passing out cigars the morning after the birth of their child. I on the other hand was shuttling back and forth from ICU and getting an education on the causes of Bell's Palsy. Oh well, the whole experience from day one had been a struggle, so why should it get any easier now? "Press on", in the immortal words of Calvin Coolidge.

That night the hospital hosted a dinner reception for all the couples who had become parents. Sort of a sterile, yet intimate, attempt to connect father and mother for a romantic meal. Lobster and Iced Tea, flowers and photos. Well, there we were, the talk of the dining room. My wife who was masquerading as Popeye, and I with a three day beard growth, bags under my eyes from exhaustion, and a wrinkled flannel shirt I had slept in the night before. I can't remember a more

197

romantic evening!

As the days passed we got better at our routines. Deb eventually went home and her face started to slowly defrost. Madison was making turtle speed progress, but it was progress. We would call or visit separately during the day and then visit together every evening after I came home from work. I always had a knot in my throat as we walked down the long winding hall, following the yellow line to where all the preemies were. How was she? Did anything happen since I last spoke to the nurse? We would walk in, store her bottles in the refrigerator, wash our hands, put on our greens, and race for her incubator. Deb would always pull her chart to see what kind of clinical progress she made that day. After talking to the nurse on duty, we would bathe her, weigh her, feed her, dress her in jammies, and then rock her to sleep. Her weight progress would come in ounces. She needed to hit five pounds before she could be discharged. It would finish up, being 22 days before she hit that plateau. Of course during the three weeks we had our ups and downs. Fevers, diarrhea, weight loss, infection, tests, lack of appetite, more tests, consultations, questions, specialists and yet more tests. When can we please get off the roller coaster? All we wanted to do was take our baby home and live a normal life. They say that adversity builds character in the individual and further bonds couples that love each other. Well I felt that I was overloaded with character, and that Deb and I were crazy glued! The reality was that our marriage kept getting stronger because of our journey. We are two very determined people, and we were going to find a way to survive this as well.

Finally, the day arrived. The kid had hit just shy of five pounds and after conflicting opinions from within the hospital staff we were given the green light to take her home. The last week she had made steady progress, and by then we were comfortable with the routine. I felt like I was even getting to "know" her. She had a personality that was unique even at that early age. I was getting to know her likes, her dislikes, her habits. She had been in good, secure hands since the day she was born and I was very "okay" with that. She had constant monitoring, a floor full of doctors, nurses, machines, and anything she needed. But now we had to break the cord again. It was time to go home. Deb was ready! The hospital said Madison was ready! The problem was that maybe DaDa was not ready! What if something happened? What if she got sick again? Was five pounds really enough? Despite all my inner apprehension and anxiety, I helped strap her into the portable car seat/ carrier, waved good-bye to all the nurses, put on my best smile and headed for home. I think I drove 12 miles per hour all the way home with my eyes fixed on the rear view mirror watching my wife and daughter's every move. My daughter...I still could not believe the sound of those words.

Chapter Fourteen
Miracle Baby Comes Home

She Said...

We were so excited to finally be bringing Madison home and so thankful that everything had turned out beautifully. We packed the baby into the back seat of that tiny Honda and I jumped (as best I could!) in there with her. From that day forward, until she was 20 pounds, I rode in the back seat of the car with her. If I had to go out and take the baby with me, I would make Shannon or Buddy come with me so they could ride in the back with her.

"Going home" day was the best! Eli drove like an old lady and I was scared to death that someone was going to slam into us because we were going too slow. Every few minutes he'd ask, "How's she doing . . . is she all right?" It was so funny to see how nervous he was. I could see the relief on his face when we finally pulled into our driveway.

Before going into the house, I showed Madison her welcome home sign and told her all about her new home. Eli was practically pushing me into the house.

"Show her later . . . get her inside before she gets cold!" It was a gorgeous, balmy Florida day! There was no way she was going to get cold. Silly daddy!

I changed her and gave her to her dad who promptly sat in the rocking chair with her and said: "Now what?" He had such a helpless look on his face.

"Now what do we do?" he asked me.

I laughed. "What do you mean what do we do? We take care of her, silly."

Eli had to leave for his appointment so that meant I had the baby all to myself. Pure luxury. It was the first time I was completely alone with her. It was wonderful. I held her close, cuddling her tiny little neck while breathing in that beautiful new baby smell. If only we could bottle that smell . . . we'd make a fortune.

When Eli came home, he found Mom and baby sound asleep on the couch.

It was strange to hear her little meowing cry and yet it was soothing. The first few weeks tested our nerves through and through. One or the other of us was constantly checking on her. I could always tell when Eli was checking her breathing. He would gently place his palm on her back and wait to feel the up and down motion and then he would lean over her cradle and kiss her cheek.

We would jump at her slightest movement. "Quick, get her, she's moving," my husband would yell. I would run to make sure she was all right. We started getting used to her being home and could recognize her demands for hunger or diapie changes. Once we felt confident that nothing was going to happen to her, we calmed down enough to enjoy her.

The kids were funny to watch also. During the first week or so, Buddy didn't want to hold her. He was afraid he would drop her. Fine with me. He would sit on the floor, next to her cradle, and just stare at her. We have pictures of Buddy's back! He didn't pick her up until she was almost three months old.

Shannon, on the other hand, couldn't wait to get her hands on her. But, little did I know I had accidentally prevented her from picking her up and indulging in being a big sister. The day we arrived home, I told Shannon: "Listen, no offense, but I don't want anyone picking her up and spreading germs. So, please tell your friends that they can see her . . . but no touching yet."

I had no idea that Shannon thought SHE was included in that warning. She would sit in the rocking chair by the baby's cradle and rock the cradle and sing softly to her, but she never picked her up. I thought it was strange for Shannon but maybe she was scared. After all the baby was only five pounds . . . so tiny!

One Saturday morning, about two weeks after we brought Madison home, I asked Shannon if she would mind keeping an eye on the baby while I took a shower.

"No problem, Mom, but what do I do if she wakes up?" she asked.

"Pick her up!" I told her. "But, you said no one was allowed to pick her up yet."

"That didn't include YOU!" I said in wonderment. "YOU can pick her up . . . just not your friends."

I couldn't believe it. She had been torturing herself for no reason! I went into my bedroom for a moment and came back out and Shannon had the baby in her arms. "What happened?" I asked. "She moved and I thought she was waking up so I picked her up," she said with a stupid grin on her face.

She sat and held that baby for hours that Saturday morning!

Everyone wanted to come and visit and see the newest little Franco. I really didn't want anyone to see my Palsy, and besides that, we were paranoid that someone might have germs and Madison would get sick! With the exception of our family, we held people off for about a month, at which time, the Palsy was doing much better.

The word was out. It was all right to visit the Franco's! They came in droves. "We were in the neighborhood . . . thought we'd stop by," said Joan and Armando who live a solid 45 minutes south of us! "I wanted to see this miracle kid before she went to college," Judy teased.

"Gee, she looks just like Eli," Janet said.

"She's got the Franco eyes," Rebeca and Rafa laughed.

"She's so precious, so tiny," Beverly said as she handed me a beautiful porcelain doll.

"She sure is some special baby; she looks just like you, Eli," Wayne repeated.

All right. So, we put the kid on display for the world to see. We smiled from ear to ear and accepted everyone's congratulations. But, it wasn't long before I started to get sick of hearing: "She looks like YOU, ELI!"

I guess almost all my wishes came true. She certainly did, and does, look like her Daddy. She has his huge, almond shaped brown eyes, and his beautiful mouth. She got my hair and skin tones and a beautiful little button nose she inherited from the Italian side of the family. She's gorgeous! But, then I think all three of my kids are beautiful! Spoken like a true mom!

In order to really make Madison's debut official, we had to present her to Dr. David and Dr. Wayne. We wanted them to witness the results of their endeavors and to savor the happy moments that result from their work!

We called and made an appointment to visit them on a Tuesday afternoon. We dressed the baby up in a little white angelic outfit and told her we were going "bye-bye" to visit some very special people. When we arrived, the nurses came out to the waiting room to giggle and coo over the baby. Everyone was so happy for us. Hugs, kisses and even a few tears were exchanged. And then Dr. David came out to see our miracle baby. Dr. Wayne had an emergency and wasn't available to see us. He took her from me without hesitation, took one look at her and said, "She looks just like this guy," pointing to Eli! I was laughing because even if I didn't already know it, I had been told it so many times, I would have no choice but to believe it!

"You know, Dr. David, Eli was afraid you might screw up and give us the wrong embryo so it's a good thing the baby looks like him," I told him laughingly.

With a smile on his face, Dr. David was shaking his fist at Eli. Both men then stepped forward and shook hands. My husband sincerely thanked him for all he had done to help us get our precious bundle.

When we left the office there were several couples waiting to see the doctor. My eyes connected with a young woman who glanced up at me, and as I smiled at her, my eyes said, "Have hope, don't give up!"

Dreams do come true.

And so do miracles.

Epilogue

She Said…

And here we are 14 years later. You must be asking yourself WHY haven't they published this book sooner? Trust me, we've asked ourselves the same question. I guess life just got away from us. Too busy climbing corporate ladders, acquiring new houses, toys, and 'stuff.' Oh yeah, we were on a roll.

Let me bring you up to date.

Ten years ago, a bigger company swallowed up Eli's company and that company made us an offer we couldn't refuse. "Move to Tampa young man, join our corporate team." Oh yeah baby, we were ready to get out of the Ft. Lauderdale area and Tampa sounded like the place to be. We packed up the house and our little girl and hit the road. Once in Tampa, we built our dream house. We were in heaven… almost 4000 square feet of Francodom. We put our pool table in and furnished the house with big screen TVs and lots of goodies. We loved it. We found a Montessori school for Madison and she thrived in the environment. Life went on. Eli kept racking up the years at his company while I found a job as Director of Marketing for a housing developer. All was well.

So, let me give you an update on the kids. Shannon married Wes, the love of her life five years ago and promptly moved two streets over from us! I just knew she would make her way to Tampa eventually. She is an assistant Vice President at a local bank and is planning on making me a grandmother soon. I'm so proud of her and her accomplishments.

After completing a four-year stint in the army, Buddy came home and met his significant other. They made me a grandmother seven years ago. My grandbaby, Kassidy, is smart, funny, and beautiful. She looks just like her daddy with her beautiful long, curly blonde hair. Buddy adores his daughter and I'm so proud of the man he has become. The family lives in Melbourne, about two hours away from me.

Ah, my Madison. She got the best of both of us. I tell her that all the time. Her personality is the best…smart, sassy, funny, intuitive, sensitive, loving, and kind. We moved her to a private school and she excelled. Straight A student, outstanding athlete…even though she's petite. She plays all sports including basketball! She is in National Junior Honor Society, participates in various clubs at her school, is crazy about boys, music and her friends. She's your typical young lady getting ready for high school.

I can't believe how the years have flown by. Great years, happy years. Until 2006. Now that year couldn't have flown by fast enough for us. July, 2006 was monumental. After 29 years with his company, Eli was laid off. "WHAT?" I said when he came home that night, in shock. I couldn't believe it. Neither could he. After a few days of shock we sprang into action. He needed a resume; he needed to know how to look for a job. He needed a boost to his ego. I was so worried about him…he wasn't the same guy. He didn't laugh, he lost weight, and he worried about everything. Luckily the company gave him a parachute, but still, he needed a job. His self worth, his ego, his everything was tied to his job. There was no laughter in our home.

August, 2006 was monumental. My breast cancer came back. Ten years ago I was diagnosed with breast cancer and had a mastectomy. After that I took tamoxifen for five years and since I didn't have any additional signs of the cancer returning, we figured that was it. Gone. Wrong. We had to deal with it again.

Friends, relatives, even strangers rallied to support us. I received tons and tons of cards, books, gifts, flowers, fruit, hats (lots of hats!) from everyone. The outpouring of love was overwhelming. I thought that with all the prayers being sent up to heaven on my behalf, I surely couldn't lose this one! I started my own marketing campaign: BELIEVE. Believe in ME and my strength, Believe in the power of prayer, and Believe that God will be generous. I told EVERYONE about my Believe campaign. Before I knew it, all my family, my friends, my doctors were believing. Ya gotta Believe!

My brother flew down from New York to take care of this family because no one was functioning very well. My sister-in-law flew down to take care of the family the next month. CHEMO, the doctor said. Once every three weeks for three months. Heck, I could handle that. No problem. Well, a little bit, but it was manageable. After the three months, we did the scans. It's not gone. Not a bit. There is no cure. They can only stabilize so the tumors don't grow.

The doctor said I had to do more...eight more weeks this time, once a week. Hard to Believe. We moped, screamed, cried, cursed, slept, and prayed. I finally said enough: Cancer is not going to run my life. BELIEVE was back!

And, that's where we are right now. In the middle of chemo. But, I BELIEVE! Oh yeah, Eli found a comparable job after only five months of being unemployed. One item off the wish list! So, since I'm not working, NOW I have time to finish the book.

We've learned so much through both of these experiences. Things that we knew but forgot. It's not the toys and goodies that mean the most in your life. It's not the expensive dinners, the drawers full of jewelry or the fancy cars that matter. It's your family that counts and we couldn't have made it through some of the tougher moments if it weren't for my brother and sister-in-law, my daughters and my son. And, Wes too!

It's your friends surrounding you with love and an available ear that matters. Thank you to all our friends who Believe and continue to cheer and pray for us. There are so many of you that I would need to write another book just to list everyone. Just know that we so appreciate each and every one of you! I am so grateful for Peg, Nikki and Pam, who have lent their shoulders to cry on and their arms to provide great big hugs. They have been my taxi drivers, providers of a good cup of coffee when it was desperately needed and chocolate to chase away the blues.

And to my forever friends who went through IVF with us, the first round of cancer, and now the second…Thank you for the laughter and Believing in me… Janet, Judy, Beca and Lorna… I love you guys.

He Said…

It's been awhile since "He" said anything. Alot has happened in 14 years. The hair is alot thinner and whiter, and there are a few more character lines on the ol' mug. We moved from the east coast to the west coast of Florida in 1997 after our company got bought out. While many of my friends and colleagues were being marched out the door, I actually got promoted with a chance to start a new life in a new city. New friends, new business associates, new everything. I loved it. Although my career really took off, the atmosphere of working for a publicly traded company was very different. The nine years in Tampa was a learning experience and very good for us financially, but the price to pay was dear. After the company made some bad investments in 2001, and after several subsequent down sizings, I lived in constant fear of the infamous corporate ax. The final three years that I worked there were no fun. Revolving bosses, constant rumors, no direction.

In July, 2006 the ax finally came. Mr Franco, thank you for

213

29 years. In exchange for an amicable separation, here is a chunk of money. Have a nice life! And just like that I was gone! Now what? I haven't looked for a job in three decades. Then, 48 days later lightning struck again. "Mrs. Franco, it looks like your breast cancer has come back." Wow, a twofer! Life is different these days. Gone are the days of traveling three to four days a week for work, and living the high life. I am now a government employee. The pace is slower because that's how government works. I'm working with a great group of down to earth people. I'm home every night so I can be engaged while Madison gets through the next couple of critical years. My wife is slowly getting her strength back and I am so grateful that I have been able to be around while she recovers. I am learning a new business, and because my job requires me to manage media relations, I am logging plenty of airtime on local television and radio, as well as print. I'm enjoying my job for the first time in a long time.

I am a different guy from the one in Chapter One. I'm a little more mellow, a little more humble and alot more thankful for the things I have. I cannot thank Debbie enough for twisting my arm one last time and making me go through IVF again.

Madison is the sunshine in my life. She has grown up to be a beautiful young lady. A student and sports jock with a sense of humor alot like her old man. She is one special kid and she has made my life wonderfully complete!